ESSENTIALS OF

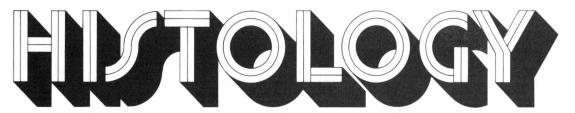

BY

Jack D. Burke Ph.D.
Professor of Anatomy, School of Basic
Sciences and Graduate Studies,
Medical College of Virginia,
Health Sciences Division of Virginia
Commonwealth University, Richmond,
Virginia.

Richard J. Weymouth PhD., M.D.
Professor of Anatomy, Lecturer of Internal
Medicine

Hugo R. Seibel Ph.D.
Associate Professor of Anatomy

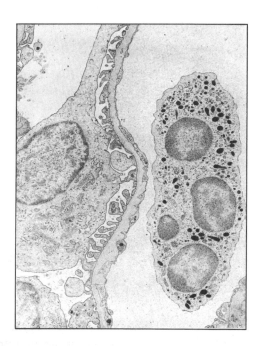

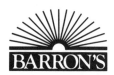

BARRON'S EDUCATIONAL SERIES, INC.

Woodbury, New York / London / Toronto / Sydney

Cover: Electron micrograph of a kidney podocyte (left), basement membrane, capillary endothelium, and a polymorphonu-
clear leukocyte in capillary lumen.

All inquiries should be addressed to:
Barron's Educational Series, Inc.
113 Crossways Park Drive
Woodbury, New York 11797

Library of Congress Catalog Card No. 75-174346

International Standard Book No. 0-8120-0439-6

PRINTED IN THE UNITED STATES OF AMERICA

4567   510   987654

Contents

Illustrations

PREFACE

Essentials of Histology is a summary outline of a course of study in histology. In no way is it intended that this syllabus be regarded as a textbook. Rather, it is to be used as an aid in both lectures and laboratories. We believe that the contents in the syllabus covers and summarizes essential information which one ordinarily presents in a formal course in histology. We have used photomicrographs to illustrate material in various cells and tissues which we think is essential in helping a student to learn histology. We made the photomicrographs from our histology loan collection.

Essentials of Histology may be useful to anyone studying histology. Not only is it suggested for an undergraduate course in histology, but the approach employed by the authors makes it useful as well for the professional student in medicine, dentistry and graduate education.

Acknowledgments: We wish to thank several people at the Medical College of Virginia for their aid; Juan A. Astruc, M.D., Ph.D., kindly criticised and offered comments on the Nerve Tissue; George W. Burke, Jr., D.D.S., advised specifically on the content and outline of the oral cavity and salivary glands; Walter J. Geeraets, M.D., generously gave us the slides from which the photomicrographs of the eye were made. And our gratitude is especially given to Mrs. Jack D. Burke for typing the manuscript so many times, and serving as art-graphic illustrator. However, any error, or correction needed, is the responsibility of the authors.

Jack D. Burke, Ph.D.
Richard J. Weymouth, M.D., Ph.D.
Hugo R. Seibel, Ph.D.

I. ANATOMY OF A CELL

I. BODY COMPONENTS

A. Body fluids

1. Vascular systems
    a. Blood
    b. Lymph
2. Intercellular fluid
3. Intracellular fluid
    a. Protoplasm
        (1) solvent: continuous phase
        (2) solute: dispersed phase
        (3) molecular solution
        (4) colloidal solution
    b. Colloids
    c. Macromolecules
        (1) polysaccharides
        (2) proteins
        (3) nucleic acids
    d. Salts
    e. Lipids
    f. Minerals
    g. Properties
        (1) irritability
        (2) conductivity
        (3) respiration
        (4) absorption
        (5) secretion
        (6) excretion
        (7) growth
        (8) reproduction
        (9) metabolism

B. Intercellular substance

1. Supports cells
2. Types in histology
    a. Formed
        (1) *examples*: collagen and elastin
    b. Amorphous ground substance
        (1) mucopolysaccharides

C. Cells

1. Components
    a. Cytoplasm
        (1) cell (*plasma*) membrane
        (2) endoplasmic reticulum
        (3) ribosomes
        (4) Golgi complex

     (5) centrosome, two centrioles
     (6) mitochondria
     (7) lysosomes
     (8) fibrils
     (9) microtubules
    (10) pinocytotic vesicles
    (11) inclusions
        (a) proteins
        (b) fats
        (c) carbohydrates
        (d) granules
        (e) pigments
        (f) crystals

b. Nucleus
    (1) nuclear membranes (*nuclear envelope*)
    (2) nuclear sap (*karyoplasm*)
    (3) nuclear chromatin (*chromosomes*)
    (4) nucleolus

II. LIGHT MICROSCOPE

A. Calibration

1. For each combination of ocular lens, body tube, and objective lens a calibration must be made. The procedure is as follows:
  a. Insert an ocular micrometer disc (*dimension in mm.*) into the ocular either below or between the lenses.
  b. Place a stage micrometer (*whose dimension is also in mm.*) on the stage of the microscope, and focus on the stage micrometer scale.
  c. Move the stage micrometer until its zero line subtends the zero line of the ocular micrometer disc.
  d. Read across the superimposed scales to any two lines which are coincident with each other.
2. Magnification factor: Divide the scale reading on the stage micrometer into the scale reading of the ocular micrometer disc.
3. Size of object:
  a. Place a histology slide on the stage of the microscope.
  b. Measure the dimension of the object on the scale of the ocular micrometer disc.
  c. Divide the Magnification Factor into the measurement obtained from the ocular micrometer disc scale: This final and actual dimension is usually stated in microns.

B. Electron Micrographs

1. Ordinarily, in the legend for a published electron micrograph, the magnification is given. Then the size of the object shown in the micrograph can be determined as follows: (*in*

measurements where the object is less than 0.1 μ, the dimen-
sions are usually given in angstrom units = Å).

2.   Object size (Å) = size (mm.) x 10^7 / magnification.

Table of Measurements

1 m = 100 cm   1 m = 3.281 ft.

1 cm = 10 mm   1 ft = 0.305 m

1 mm = 1000 μ   1 cm = 0.394 in.

1 μ = 10,000 Å   1 in = 2.540 cm

1 mμ = 10 Å

4

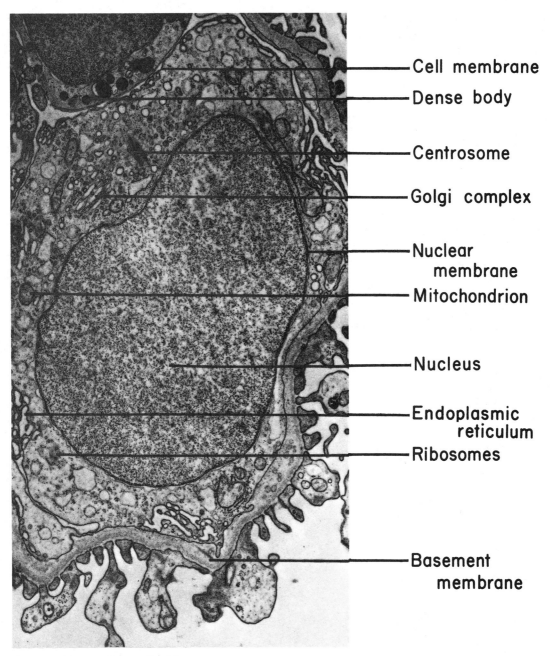

Cell membrane

Dense body

Centrosome

Golgi complex

Nuclear membrane

Mitochondrion

Nucleus

Endoplasmic reticulum

Ribosomes

Basement membrane

Anatomy of a Cell

I. MICROSCOPY

    A. Microscopes are usually classified according to the type of light source. Besides the (*visible*) light (LM) and electron (EM) microscopes, there are others such as polarization, phase contrast, interference, ultraviolet, and x-ray microscopes.

II. STAINS

    A. Dyes are used in solution to stain generally, nucleus and/or cytoplasm, or specifically, particular cellular components. Various stains usually require special fixation and tissue preparation.

    B. Dyes: neutral salts having both acidic and basic radicals

        1. Basic dye: Coloring property is in the basic radical of the neutral salt. Structures so stained are basophilic; for instance, nucleus.
        2. Acidic dyes: Staining property is in the acidic radical of the neutral salt. Structures so stained are acidophilic; for instance, cytoplasm.

    C. Examples

        1. Hematoxylin stains nuclei blue.
        2. Iron hematoxylin stains chromosomes, mitochondria, Golgi complex, and contractile elements of muscle cells black or dark blue.
        3. Carmine stains nuclei red - purple.
        4. Basic aniline dyes, such as toluidine blue, azure A and methylene blue stain mucopolysaccharides metachromatically; others also in common use are neutral red, Janus green, and brilliant cresyl blue.
        5. Acidic dyes, such as eosin, picric acid, acid azo dyes (*such as chromotrope*), and acid diazo dyes (*as trypan blue and trypad red*) stain the general cytoplasm.
        6. The common histological stain is hematoxylin and eosin.
        7. Mallory's connective tissue (CT) stain and the Mallory-Azan method stain collagen fibers bright blue, nuclei red or orange, and various cell components blue, red, orange, or purple.
        8. Masson's trichrome method stains CT green, nuclei blue or purple, and cytoplasmic structures red.
        9. Reticular fibers are stained brown by silver impregnation methods (*argyrophilic*). Reticular fibers are continuous with collagenous fibers, and are not as easily seen with H & E as collagenous fibers. Elastic fibers do not stain well with H & E, but selectively stain with orcein (*brown*) and resorcin fuchsin (*dark blue or purple*).

III. SECTION TECHNIQUE

    A. Histology slides are prepared for study by making sections. A
        section is a (*ca. 5* μ) slice of tissue fixed flat on a glass
        slide, stained, mounted in a medium of proper refractive index,
        and covered with a coverglass. Most sections are prepared by the
        paraffin method.

    B. Paraffin method - General

        1. Fixation
            a. A piece of fresh tissue is placed in a killing and fixing
                fluid such as a solution of formalin, picric acid, osmic
                acid, mercury bichloride, potassium dichromate, ethyl
                alcohol, or Bouin's fluid or other mixtures.
        2. Dehydration
            a. Ordinarily, water is removed from the tissue by passing it
                through a series of ethyl alcohol solutions of increasing
                concentrations to absolute alcohol.
        3. Clearing
            a. Although water and alcohol are not soluble in paraffin,
                substances (*called clearing agents*) such as xylol, toluol,
                chloroform, benzene, and cedar oil are soluble in both
                alcohol and melted paraffin. The tissue is taken from
                absolute alcohol and placed in the clearing agent.
        4. Embedding
            a. The tissue is placed in melted paraffin which is replaced
                with fresh wax at intervals. Finally, the tissue is
                hardened by cooling in a block of paraffin which may be
                stored indefinitely.
        5. Cutting sections
            a. The paraffin block containing the tissue is affixed to a
                microtome, and a ribbon of thin sections (*ca. 5* μ *thick*)
                sliced off. Some of these are cemented to a glass slide
                with a substance like albumin, and flattened with the aid
                of a drop of water and heat. Slides are then dried for a
                few hours in an oven.
        6. Staining
            a. The slide is now placed in the clearing agent to dissolve
                out the paraffin, and then in absolute alcohol to remove
                the clearing agent, and down a series of alcohol solutions
                to water. After staining with an aqueous solution (*of
                hematoxylin*), the slide is passed through an ascending
                series of alcohols to the clearing agent. The coverslip
                is then attached with a mounting medium, such as
                Permount.

C. Paraffin method - Specific

1. Preparation of reagents for killing and fixation.
    a. Buffered neutral formalin solution

            40% formaldehyde 100   ml.
            distilled water 900   ml.
            sodium phosphate (*monobasic*)   4   gm.
            sodium phosphate dibasic (*anhydrous*) ..   6.5 gm.

2. Preparation of reagents for staining:
    a. Hematoxylin is a chromogen derived from logwood, *Hematoxy-
        lin campechianum*, and is one of the most important of all
        stains. The dye solution itself has little or no affinity
        for tissues unless iron or aluminum is present in the
        latter; consequently *mordanting* in some form is necessary.
        The stain is made up in combination or in conjunction with
        various metallic salts.
    b. Harris's hematoxylin solution

            hematoxylin crystals ....   5.0 gm.
            alcohol, absolute ....   50.0 ml.
            ammonium (*or potassium*) alum ...... 100.0 gm.
            distilled water .... 1000.0 ml.
            mercuric oxide (*red*) ....   2.5 gm.

        Dissolve the hematoxylin in the alcohol.
        Dissolve the alum in water using heat.
        Remove from heat and mix the two solutions. Boil quickly.
        Remove from heat and add the mercuric oxide slowly. Re-
          heat the solution until it turns dark purple. Remove
          the vessel and cool in a basin of cold water. Add 3 ml.
          glacial acetic acid per 100 ml. hematoxylin solution.
          Filter.

    c. *Eosin solution*

            Eosin Y. water soluble .... 10.0 gm.
            potassium dichromate ....   5.0 gm.
            picric acid, saturated aqueous ..... 100.0 ml.
            alcohol, absolute .... 100.0 ml.
            distilled water .... 800.0 ml.

3. Cleaning slides and glassware: DO NOT SPILL ON HANDS

    a. potassium dichromate .... 20 gm.
        distilled water .... 100 ml.
        concentrated sulphuric acid .... 100 ml.

Dissolve the dichromate in the water, add the acid CAUTIOUSLY in small amounts, and cool the mixture between each addition of acid. The mixture must be stored in glass containers and may be used repeatedly until it becomes dark. Immerse the glassware for a few hours, and wash thoroughly in running water, finally rinsing with distilled water. IF THIS SOLUTION IS SPILLED, WASH IMMEDIATELY WITH COLD WATER.

4. Mayer's albumin adhesive:

Beat the white of an egg and pour it into a cylinder. Let stand until the air brings all suspended matter to the top. Skim off the latter and to the remainder add an equal volume of glycerin, and a few crystals of thymol as a preservative.

5. Dehydration
   a. Place small pieces of tissues in the killing and fixing fluid for 20-24 hours. After fixation, wash the tissues in several changes of 50% alcohol and in 70% alcohol. Dehydration is continued by removing the tissue from the vial and placing it in 95% alcohol and then into 100% alcohol. Allow tissue to remain two hours in each solution.

6. Clearing
   a. The tissue is transferred to benzene for clearing. This step makes the tissue transparent.

7. Embedding
   a. After the tissue has been cleared in the benzene small chips of paraffin are dropped into the container. It is then placed in the oven set at about 56-58° for 4-6 hours. As evaporation continues, small chips of paraffin may be added. Place the tissue in a change of melted paraffin. Remove some melted paraffin from the oven and pour a little of it into the mold. Allow the paraffin to harden somewhat, place the tissue on it, and cover the tissue with melted paraffin. As soon as a crust has formed on the paraffin, immerse the block in a beaker of cold water. The tissue is now ready for sectioning.

8. Cutting section
   a. The paraffin block is attached to a microtome device and inserted into the proper niche of a microtome. Sections are usually cut at 6-10 microns in thickness for ordinary tissues. A small camel-hair brush is useful in taking the ribbon of paraffin off the knife edge.
   b. Float the sections in a warm water bath.
   c. Take a clean slide and add a very small drop of the albumin adhesive to it. Wipe this drop over the middle surface of the slide where the cut section is to be placed. Place the section on the slide and air dry. Oven-dry overnight.

9. Staining
   a. Grease the top of several Coplin jars with vaseline. Into the jars place the following solutions:

Xylene; 1/2 xylene and 1/2 100% alcohol; 100% alcohol; 95% alcohol; 80% alcohol; 70% alcohol; 50% alcohol; 35% alcohol; distilled water; tap water; eosin stain; and hematoxylin stain.

b. Pass the slide into the xylene, then to the 1/2 xylene and 1/2 100% alcohol, to the 95, 80, 70, 50, 35% alcohol, and finally into the distilled water. The slide is then put into the hematoxylin stain for a few minutes; if over-staining occurs, de-stain in water that has had about four drops of hydrochloric acid added to it. The slide is then rinsed in tap water, dipped in an aqueous saturated solution of lithium carbonate, and passed to the distilled water, 35, 50, 70, 80% alcohol. Counter-staining is now done with the eosin in 95% alcohol for a few seconds. The slide is then taken to the 95 and 100% alcohol, into the half xylene and half alcohol mixture, and then deposited in the xylene jar. The cover-slip is now ready to be attached.

c. The slide is removed from the xylene, a drop of Permount is put on the tissue, the cover-slip is then placed over the tissue. The slide is placed in an oven to dry.

IV. HISTOCHEMISTRY

A. Since tissues are composed of various chemicals such as proteins, carbohydrates, lipids, inorganic salts and miscellaneous substances, various tests are used for their detection.

B. Examples

1. Proteins (*with tyrosine*) - yellow color
2. Enzymes - various tests for phosphatases, lipases, oxidases, esterases, and dehydrogenases.
3. Carbohydrates - glycogen by periodic acid Schiff test results in a magenta or purple color; glycoproteins give a positive PAS magenta color, but are amylase-resistant. Basement membranes and reticular fibers (*but not collagenous and elastic*) are strongly PAS positive.
4. Lipids - Sudan dyes or osmic acid
5. Inorganic salts - microincineration
6. Nucleic acids - Feulgen reaction is specific for DNA, but not for RNA, which can be detected by ribonuclease. Both DNA and RNA are basophilic.

C. Electron Microscopy - General

1. Fixation
   a. Tissues should be fixed as promptly and as rapidly as possible. Tissue blocks should be cut of such thickness

that they will not exceed 1 mm^3; the volume of fixative employed should be adequate. Osmium tetroxide and/or glutaraldehyde are commonly employed.

b. All fixatives should be carefully prepared in a hood to avoid prolonged breathing of harmful vapors. Fixatives should be stored, preferably in brown ground glass stop-pered bottles, in the refrigerator. Fixation should be carried out in the refrigerator at 0-4° C, with the fixa-tion vial resting in a dish of ice water. Fixation times vary from 1/2 to 2 hours in the case of osmium tetroxide, and from 1 to 4 hours in the case of glutaraldehyde. Glutaraldehyde fixation is usually followed by one hour of osmium tetroxide post-fixation.

2. Dehydration

a. After the tissue blocks have been properly fixed, dehydra-tion is achieved by passing the specimen through a graded series of ethyl alcohol or acetone in increasing concen-trations to absolute alcohol; the purpose of dehydration is to remove all the free water from the specimen and to replace it with ethyl alcohol or acetone, since the embed-ding media are not miscible with water.

b. Usually after glutaraldehyde fixation, the tissue samples are briefly washed in a buffer employed to remove any ex-cess fixative. In the laboratory, tissue is usually de-hydrated by passing it through 50, 75, and 95% alcohols, allowing between 5 to 10 minutes in each. The final de-hydration in absolute alcohol is usually carried out in three changes of fifteen minutes each.

3. Embedding

a. After the last change in absolute alcohol it is most de-sirable to employ an intermediate solvent between the dehydrating agent and the embedding material. Agents used as intermediate solvents are propylene oxide, xylene, toluene, acetone and styrene.

b. The purpose of embedding is to place the tissues in a solid medium that will provide sufficient strength to ob-tain thin sections. Embedding agents commonly employed are: Araldite, Epon, Maraglas, D.E.R., Vestopal W., and Durcupan.

c. Infiltration of the fixed and dehydrated tissue usually is accomplished overnight. Tissues and agents for polymeri-zation are usually placed in gelatin capsules, beem capsules or various kinds of flat embedding devices and left in an oven at 37° to 60° C, for 1 to 2 days.

4. Sectioning

a. Block trimming: The resin with the embedded tissue is trimmed until the tissue block has an exposed trapezoidal face of about 0.5 mm. Trimming may be done initially with a razor blade and then completed using a glass knife in the microtome.

  b. The sequences after this phase are: mounting the block in
      the microtome chuck, breaking and selecting a knife,
      trough or boat preparation, adjustment of binocular micro-
      scope, orientation and alignment of knife and block face,
      adjusting illumination and filling the trough with flota-
      tion fluid. Sections of approximately 600 Å in thickness
      are then obtained and placed on copper grids.

5. Staining
  a. Specimens are stained for electron microscopy to enhance
      the contrast of a section to be examined. In fact, stain-
      ing sections for electron microscopic examination results
      in the addition of heavy atoms to the specimen, which help
      in the scattering of electrons and thereby increase the
      final contrast of the section. While many attempts have
      been made, good stains for specific substances are still
      lacking, but the general staining that is carried out is
      extremely helpful to the investigator. While in most
      cases only thin sections are stained, staining can be
      carried out during fixation and dehydration.

D. Electron microscopy - Specific

1. Fixation
  a. The fixative must modify the cell to resist further treat-
      ments and also to make further treatments possible. Fixa-
      tives may be classified as either coagulant or non-coagu-
      lant. Examples of each are:
      (1) coagulant
           (a) methanol
           (b) ethanol
           (c) acetone
           (d) nitric acid
           (e) hydrochloric acid
           (f) picric acid
           (g) trichloroacetic acid
           (h) mercuric chloride
      (2) non-coagulant
           (a) formaldehyde
           (b) glutaraldehyde
           (c) osmium tetroxide
           (d) potassium dichromate
           (e) acetic acid
           (f) potassium permanganate
  b. Fixatives can also be subclassified into two categories
      and examples are listed below.
      (1) additive
           (a) osmium tetroxide
           (b) formaldehyde
           (c) glutaraldehyde

        (2) <u>non-additive</u>
- (a) methanol
- (b) ethanol
- (c) acetone

c. Common fixatives are:

(1) Palade's buffered osmium tetroxide fixative.
Prepare:

(a) veronal-acetate buffer

sodium veronal (*barbital sodium*)	1.47 gm
sodium acetate	0.97 gm

dilute to 50 ml with distilled water
Keep in refrigerator; very stable buffer.

(b) 2% solution of osmium tetroxide.
1.00 gm osmium tetroxide is dissolved in 50 ml distilled water. This should be done a day in advance since osmium tetroxide takes a long time to dissolve. It is, however, quite stable and keeps for some weeks at 4°.

(c) 0.1 N Hydrochloric acid solution.
concentrated HCL - 12 N
dilute HCL - 6 N
1 N = 88 ml/liter
6 N = 528 ml/liter
To prepare 1 N HCL from 6 N, 1.7 ml 6 N and 8.3 ml distilled water should be mixed.
To prepare 0.1 N HCL from 6 N, 0.17 ml of 6 N and 9.83 ml of distilled water should be united.
To prepare 200 ml of 0.1 N HCL from 12 N, 1.6 ml of 12 N HCL and 198.4 ml of distilled water should be mixed.

(d) fixative is prepared by mixing:
25 ml of 2% osmium tetroxide
10 ml of veronal - acetate buffer
10 ml of 0.1 N HCL
5 ml distilled water

(e) adjust the pH of the buffered solution to be between 7.3 and 7.5.

(2) Caulfield's buffered osmium tetroxide fixative.
- (a) prepare Palade's fixative.
- (b) adjust pH to 7.4.
- (c) add 2.25 g of sucrose (*0.045 g/ml animals*) (*0.015 g/ml plants*).
- (d) check the pH again.

Caulfield increased the molarity of Palade's fixative.

(3) Zetterqvist's buffered isotonic osmium tetroxide fixative.
Palade's fixative is slightly hypotonic and the use of an isotonic fixative is desirable for some specimens.

Prepare:
(a) veronal-acetate buffer
(b) 2% osmium tetroxide solution
(c) the following Ringer's solution
     sodium chloride 8.05 gm
     potassium chloride 0.42 gm
     calcium chloride 0.18 gm
     Make up to 100 ml with distilled water.
(d) 0.1 N HCL solution
(e) fixative is prepared by mixing:
     25 ml of 2% osmium tetroxide
     10 ml of veronal - acetate buffer
     34 ml of Ringer's solution
     11.0 ml of 0.1 N HCL

(4) glutaraldehyde fixation.
   (a) glutaraldehyde-phosphate fixative.
      1. prepare the phosphate buffer:
          0.2M $NaH_2PO_4 \cdot H_2O$ (27.6 g/L) 23 ml
          0.2M $Na_2HPO_4 \cdot 2H_2O$ (35.61 g/L) 77 ml
          unite and dilute to 200 ml with distilled
          water to obtain a pH of 7.3.
      2. the final fixative is obtained by mixing
          12 ml of 25% glutaraldehyde and 88 ml of
          buffer.
      3. some investigators also add 10 drops of 1%
          $CaCl_2$ to a 100 ml solution of buffer.
   (b) glutaraldehyde-cacodylate fixative.
      1. this mixture is made in the following
          manner:
          25 ml of 25% glutaraldehyde
          75 ml of 0.1 M cacodylate buffer
      2. check pH and adjust to 7.4.
   (c) glutaraldehyde-veronal acetate fixative.
        Make the fixative as follows:
        12 ml of 25% glutaraldehyde
        38 ml of distilled water
        50 ml of veronal-acetate buffer
        0.24 gm of calcium chloride.
   (d) some of the criteria of good fixation are:
      1. nuclei should present a uniform and finely
          granular appearance; clumping of chromatin
          material is usually a sign of poor fixation.
      2. mitochondria should show no swelling, dis-
          ruption of their membranes or empty, washed
          out appearance.
      3. the endoplasmic reticulum should present a
          fairly uniform and distinct appearance.
      4. no disruptions or discontinuities should be
          found in the plasma membrane.

        5. the ground substance of the cytoplasm should be finely granular and exhibit no clumping or precipitations.

        6. shrinkage spaces or spaces in general should be viewed with caution; tearing of cells from other structures is a bad indication.

        7. an aesthetically pleasing picture is probably still the best criterion of good fixation.

(5) dehydration

    (a) a typical dehydration and processing schedule recommended to the beginner is outlined below:

Step		Time
*1.	fixation	
2.	washing	
3.	30% ethyl alcohol	5 minutes
4.	50% ethyl alcohol	5 minutes
5.	70% ethyl alcohol	5 minutes
6.	95% ethyl alcohol	5 minutes
7.	100% ethyl alcohol	15 minutes
8.	100% ethyl alcohol	15 minutes
9.	100% ethyl alcohol	15 minutes
10.	100% ethyl alcohol + propylene oxide (1 = 1)	5 minutes
11.	propylene oxide	15 minutes
12.	propylene oxide	15 minutes
13.	propylene oxide + embedding mixture (1:1)	1 hour
**14.	propylene oxide + embedding mixture (1:2)	2 hours
15.	embedding media	overnight
16.	embed	

*Steps 1-8 should be carried out at 4°C; the rest are carried out at room temperature.
**Step 14 may be omitted.

(6) embedding

    (a) tne properties of an ideal embedding medium are:

        1. it should be completely soluble in ethyl alcohol or acetone.

        2. it should have a low viscosity so that it may penetrate the specimen easily and completely.

        3. it should harden uniformly and without shrinkage.

        4. the block should be hard enough to allow thin sections to be cut relatively easily.

        5. sections obtained should be fairly easy to stain.

    6. sections should retain configuration and
        stability under electron bombardment.
(b) mixtures
    1. araldite
        27 ml - araldite casting resin M or 502
        23 ml - dodecenyl succinic anhydride (DDSA)
        1.5 to 2% v/v;
        added just before use - DMP - 30 accelerator
    2. epon
        a. the resin components are made up as
            follows:

Mixture A

Epon 812	62 ml	These mixtures may be
DDSA	100 ml	stored in the refrigerator
		up to 6 months. If kept

Mixture B

Epon 812	100 ml	cold, mixtures should be
MNA	89 ml	warmed past dew point
		before opening.

Mixture A ml	Mixture B ml	Total Vol. ml	Accelerator DMP - 30) ml	Equiv. Hardness Methacrylate
10	0	10	.15	100% n-butyl
7	3	10	.15	10-15% methyl
5	5	10	.15	15-20% methyl
3	7	10	.15	20-30% methyl
0	10	10	.15	30-50% methyl

    3. D.E.R. preparation.
        a. the following embedding formulas are
            advocated:

                              Mixtures
                            Volume in ml.

	1	2	3
D.E.R. 332	7	7	6
D.E.R. 732	3	2	3
DDSA	5	5	10
DMP-30 (or 10)	0.30	0.28	0.38

            mixture 1 is the softest and is recom-
            mended for tissues such as kidney, liver,
            heart, small bowel and suspensions of
            leucocytes.

mixture 2 is harder and suitable for
tissues high in collagen content.
mixture 3 is of the same hardness as 1
but stronger sections due to the high
DDSA content are obtained. D.E.R. 732
content controls the hardness .

(7) staining
  (a) procedure
    1. place a slide dipped in melted paraffin in a
        Petri dish.
    2. NaOH pellets are placed in the dish in order
        to prevent the formation of precipitates.
    3. a drop of stain is placed upon the slide
        using a pipette.
    4. grids are placed, sections facing downward,
        upon the drop of stain.
    5. the Petri dish must be kept tightly closed
        during staining.
    6. rinse the grids in a stream of distilled water.
    7. touch the grids to filter paper and allow to
        dry.
  (b) specific stains
    1. lead hydroxide
      a. prepare a nearly saturated solution of
          lead acetate by dissolving 8.26 grams
          of the lead salt in 15 ml of distilled
          water.
      b. rapidly add 3.2 ml of aqueous 40 per cent
          sodium hydroxide (NaOH).
      c. stir this mixture vigorously and centri-
          fuge it.
      d. discard supernatant and resuspend the
          material again in an equal amount of
          distilled water.
      e. centrifuge and discard supernatant parti-
          cles and resuspend as above.
      f. centrifuge and discard supernatant and
          resuspend as above.
      g. store at room temperature.
      h. stain from 1 - 45 minutes.
      i. rinse in distilled water thoroughly.
    2. lead citrate at a high pH
        The stain here differs from other alkaline
        lead stains in that the chelating agent is
        citrate. When droplets of fresh staining
        solution of alkaline lead citrate were ex-
        posed to the air for times as long as 30
        minutes, no precipitates formed.
      a. place 1.33 gm lead nitrate, 1.76 gm.
          sodium citrate and 30 ml distilled water

in a 50 ml volumetric flask. Shake
vigorously for one minute and allow to
stand with intermittent shaking.

b. after 30 minutes add 8.0 ml 1 N sodium
    hydroxide, dilute to 50 ml with distilled
    water and mix by inversion.

c. lead citrate dissolves and stain is ready
    for use. pH is usually 12.0 plus or minus
    0.1. Faint turbidity may be removed by
    centrifugation. Stain is stable for six
    months.

d. stain by placing grid section side down
    on drop of stain on wax-covered slide
    dish. Time of staining depends upon
    fixative and embedment used.

e. methacrylate material stains readily in
    5 to 10 minutes. Araldite, Maraglas or
    Epon stain in 15 to 30 minutes. Tissues
    fixed in phosphate buffered osmium
    tetroxide and glutaraldehyde stain so
    intensely that the stain is usually
    diluted 1:5 up to 1:1000 and the staining
    time reduced to five minutes.

f. following staining, grids are washed
    sequentially in jet of 0.02N sodium
    hydroxide and distilled water from plastic
    bottles and allowed to dry.

I. EPITHELIUM

    A. Cells are arranged in sheets which cover or line surfaces, or appear as cell masses in glands.

    B. Simple

        1. Squamous - Bowman's capsule of kidney.
        2. Cuboidal - tubules of kidney.
        3. Columnar - gallbladder - nonciliated.
                  - uterine tube - ciliated.

    C. Pseudostratified

        1. Columnar - male urethra - nonciliated.
                  - trachea - ciliated.

    D. Stratified

        1. Squamous - skin - keratinizing.
                  - vagina - nonkeratinizing.
        2. Cuboidal - sweat glands.
        3. Columnar - male urethra.
        4. Transitional - urinary bladder.

    E. Attachment of cells

        1. Intercellular cement.
        2. Cell web is fibrillar material which serves a supportive role within many kinds of cells. The filaments commonly are anchored to:
            a. Discoid shaped desmosomes which are electron-dense areas of the cytoplasmic membranes of adjacent cells separated by alternate dark and light lamellae.
            b. Fibrillar elements attached to the desmosomes dark areas (*attachment plaques*) are called tonofibrils.
        3. Terminal bars are thickened areas of opposing cell membranes surrounding the apical portion (*unlike desmosomes*) of the cell in a corona composed of both the tight and loose junctions.
        4. Junctional complexes have three parts indicated from the surface of a cell to its base.
            a. Zonula occludens (*tight junction*)
            b. Zonula adherens (*loose junction*)
            c. Macula adherens (*desmosome*)
        5. Basement membrane
            a. Basal lamina (*form of collagen*).
            b. Reticular fibers lie in a ground substance containing polysaccharides.

F. Specialization of the cell surface.

   1. Microvilli are tubelike evaginations of the cytoplasmic membrane containing a core of cytoplasm. They form a brush or striated border in many epithelia.
   2. Stereocilia are nonmotile, long and slender microvilli.
   3. Cilia - each cilium contains nine longitudinal peripheral and two central filaments. The "9 + 2" filaments consist of two microtubules each. This appearance is similar to that of centrioles and basal bodies, but there are only nine triplet longitudinal microtubules in the two latter organelles.

II. GLANDULAR EPITHELIUM

A. A system of either single cells or multicellular masses of epithelial cells highly specialized for secretion.

B. Exocrine

   1. Unicellular glands
     a. Goblet (*mucous*) cell - intestine and trachea
     b. Mucous cell - stomach
   2. Multicellular glands
     a. These glands consist of epithelial cells lining its duct system (*excretory ducts*), and those of its secretory units (*end pieces*) arising as a surface invagination into vascularized CT. If the duct persists, the gland is exocrine; if not, the end pieces secrete into capillaries and the gland is endocrine.
   3. Simple
     a. Tubular glands
       (1) straight - large intestine (*crypts of Lieberkühn*)
       (2) coiled - sweat glands of the skin
       (3) branched - fundic, pyloric, and cardiac glands of the stomach
     b. Alveolar glands
       (1) meibomian glands of the eyelid
       (2) sebaceous glands of the skin
     c. Tubulo-alveolar
       (1) salivary glands, Brunner's gland of the duodenum, and mucous glands of the esophagus
   4. Compound - Each of the lobules is a unit that is equivalent to a simple, branched gland.
     a. Tubular
       (1) kidney, testis
     b. Alveolar
       (1) mammary gland
     c. Tubulo-alveolar
       (1) pancreas and parotid

     5. Secretory cells - types
        a. Serous - parotid glands
        b. Mucous - palatine glands
        c. Mixed sero-mucous - mandibular and sublingual glands.
        d. Eccrine (*merocrine*) - the secretion is a product of the cell - majority of glands.
        e. Apocrine - apical ends of cells break off and form a part of the secretion - mammary gland.
        f. Holocrine - extrusion of entire cells filled with secretion - sebaceous gland.

C. Endocrine glands

(*See "Endocrine System"*)

III. FALSE EPITHELIUM   (*This epithelium is termed false in the sense that the cells are derived from mesoderm*).

A. Endothelium

    1. Lines blood vessels, heart, and lymph vessels.

B. Mesothelium

    1. Lines pleural, pericardial, and peritoneal cavities.

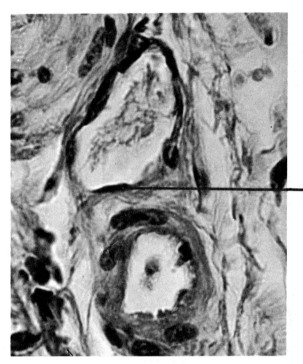 simple squamous
epithelium

Endothelium

22

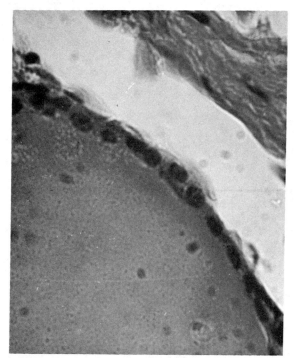

Simple cuboidal epithelium

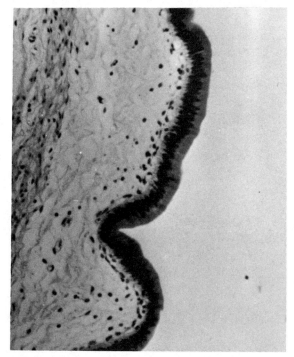

Simple columnar epithelium

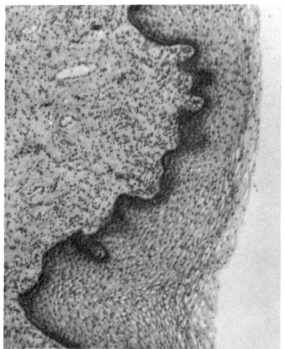

Stratified squamous epithelium

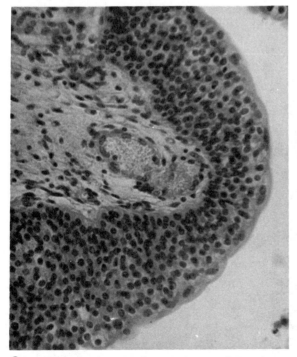

Stratified transitional epithelium

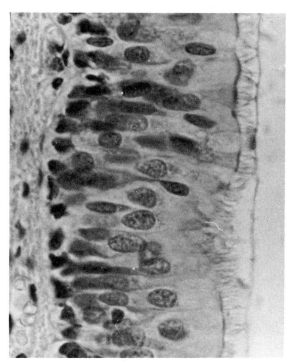

Pseudostratified ciliated columnar epithelium

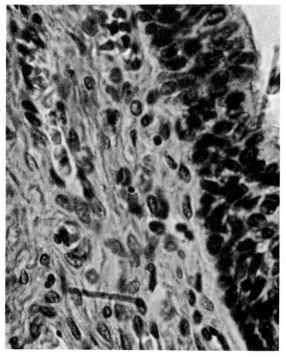

Stratified columnar epithelium

IV. CONNECTIVE TISSUE PROPER

I. COMPONENTS OF CONNECTIVE TISSUE (*CT*) PROPER

A. CT is composed of 3 elements - cells, fibers, and amorphous ground substance. The CT develops from embryonic mesenchyme. It is composed of stellate and fusiform cells which form a network, and an amorphous ground substance with scattered fibers. Mesenchymal cells have the potential to differentiate and develop along several lines to produce many different kinds of CT.

B. Cells

1. Fibroblasts
   a. These cells are considered responsible for collagenous and reticular fiber formation as well as the elaboration of the amorphous ground substance of the matrix. Mature fibroblasts (*fibrocytes*) are weakly basophilic as contrasted to young ones. Although fixed cells, upon stimulation, they become motile.
2. Undifferentiated mesenchymal cells
   a. These cells are probably similar to the primitive reticular cells seen in hemopoietic tissues. The cells are smaller than fibroblasts, usually not associated with fibers, and generally found along the walls of capillaries. They are capable of developing into various cell types.
3. Macrophages
   a. Histiocytes, or macrophages, are abundant in highly vascularized areas, and are about as numerous as fibroblasts in loose CT. They are phagocytic and are one component of the Reticuloendothelial System.
4. Fat cells
   a. Adipose tissue is formed when fat cells accumulate in large numbers. They are a normal component of areolar tissue. Fat cells are fully differentiated and do not undergo mitosis.
5. Mast cells
   a. The mast cell is characterized by the presence of metachromatic granules in the cytoplasm. Possibly they produce heparin. There is also some evidence that they produce histamine and serotonin.
6. Blood leucocytes (*see "Specialized CT: Blood"*)
   a. Lymphocytes are more numerous in the CT which supports the respiratory and alimentary tracts. They accumulate in areas of chronic inflammation, and seem to pass freely to and from the circulatory system.
   b. Eosinophils are usually plentiful in the CT of the respiratory and alimentary tracts as well as the CT of the lactating breast.
   c. Neutrophils may be seen in regions of inflammation.

        d. Plasma cells are more frequently found in serous membranes
and lymphoid tissue although they seem plentiful in chronic
inflammation. They somewhat resemble lymphocytes, and as
with lymphocytes, there is evidence that they are possible
sites of antibody formation.
        e. Pigment cells are commonly found in the skin, pia mater
and choroid coat of the eye. Because melanin is present,
they are also called melanocytes.

C. Fibers

   1. There are three kinds of fibers present in adult CT. They are
all represented in each type of CT in varying degrees.
     a. Collagenous fibers
       (1) are also called white fibers because they are color-
less in a fresh preparation.
       (2) they are the most numerous of CT fibers, and consist
of collagen, a protein. Each fiber-bundle may have
a thickness up to 100 μ, a fiber (*comprising fibrils*)
may vary from 1 to 12 μ, in D., a fibril (*comprising
microfibrils*) is about 0.4 μ thick.
       (3) microfibrils (*ca. 0.04* μ *thick*) run parallel, and are
cross-banded with a periodicity of 640 Å; they are
also birefringent in polarized light and stain pink-
red with H & E.
     b. Reticular fibers
       (1) each fiber is about 0.2 to 1 μ thick, and comprised
of fibrils whose thickness approaches that of the
collagenic microfibril.
       (2) a reticulum is formed by the uniting of branching
fibers; it is argyrophilic, and PAS positive. The
fibrous framework is formed in lymphoid and hemopoietic tissue and in basement membranes of epithelia.
       (3) reticular fibers are inelastic, but can be continuous
with collagen fibers. Reticular fibers also have a
periodic spacing of 640 Å.
     c. Elastic fibers
       (1) consist of the albuminoid elastin. The highly elastic
fibers form a network, and occur singly, not in
bundles. In the fresh state, they appear yellow.
       (2) each fiber is homogeneous, varies in diameter from
about 1 to as much as 12 μ, and will stretch to about
1.5 times the length before breaking. Selectively,
they are stained with orcein, resorsin-fuchsin, and
Verhoeff's stain.

D. Ground substance

    1. CT cells and fibers are embedded in an amorphous (*viscous or gel*) ground substance. When fresh, it is transparent and optically homogeneous, and can be preserved by freeze-drying. It is extracted by ordinary fixatives, and varies in consistency. It stains metachromatically with toluidine blue because of the mucopolysaccharides present. Evidence supports the view that fibroblast granules are the precursors of the amorphous ground substance.

II. TYPES OF CT PROPER

A. General: Although the appearance of CT depends on the arrangement and dimension of cells, fibers, and ground substance, the concentration of fibers really determines the CT type. A loose arrangement of fibers classifies a CT as Loose Connective Tissue; conversely, an abundance of fibers compactly arranged classifies a CT as Dense Connective Tissue.

    1. Loose CT
        a. Mesenchyme - embryo and fetus
            (1) cells - scanty cytoplasm, relatively large and pale nucleus, totipotential, stellate or fusiform, no true syncytium formed, smaller than fibroblasts.
            (2) fibers - fine fibrils in later stages.
            (3) ground substance - coagulable fluid in early stages, later forming a mucoid jelly.
        b. Mucous CT - Wharton's jelly of umbilical cord; otherwise it is a transient type.
            (1) cells - large stellate fibroblasts and a few macrophages and migratory lymphocytes.
            (2) fibers - a few collagenous fibers present.
            (3) ground substance - is soft and jelly-like, gives a mucin reaction, and stains with toluidine blue.
        c. Areolar CT - found in almost every microscopic section of the body as a loosely arranged fibro-elastic connective tissue (FECT).
            (1) cells - all CT cells described above; commonest are macrophages and fibroblasts.
            (2) fibers; collagenous are more abundant than elastic fibers, which, in turn, are in excess of reticular fibers found more abundantly in areas where areolar tissue borders on other structures (*as basement membranes*).
            (3) ground substance; an amorphous jelly-like coagulable fluid.

      d. Adipose tissue - areolar tissue generally holds fat cells; where these cells accumulate (*in the panniculus adiposus beneath the skin, mesentery, and bone marrow regions*) they form adipose tissue.

           (1) cells - a clear spheroid about 120 μ in diameter, highly refractive, usually containing a droplet of oil, and a thin shell of cytoplasm with a nucleus. Lobules are formed by closely packed fat cells which are separated by fibrous septa.

           (2) fibers - fine reticular fibers that surround each fat cell; the tissue spaces in the web contain fibroblasts, mast cells and eosinophils, and lymphoid cells.

           (3) ground substance - amorphous ground substance.

      e. Reticular tissue - forms framework of liver, bone marrow, and lymphoid organs.

           (1) cells - primitive reticular cells with a large pale nucleus, considerable cytoplasm that is stellate shaped, produce fibers, and resemble embryonic mesenchymal cells; larger fixed phagocytic reticular cells which can become free macrophages; other CT cells are also present.

           (2) fibers - cytoplasmic extensions envelop or extend along the fibers.

           (3) ground substance - amorphous ground substance.

2. Dense CT

      a. Dense irregular CT

           (1) interlacing fibers forming sheets with limited space for ground substance and tissue fluid. Collagenous fibers are predominant but elastic and reticular fibers are also present. Fibroblasts and some macrophages are present.

           (2) examples are most fascias, dermis of the skin, capsule of spleen and testis (*tunica albuginea*), periosteum, dura mater, and epimysium.

      b. Dense regular CT

           (1) densely packed fibers lie parallel to each other forming structures of great tensile strength.

               (a) tendon - the unit structure is a primary tendon bundle which is a large collagenous fiber; fibroblasts are aligned forming rows between bundles.

               (b) ligaments; similar in structure to tendons, but some (*ligamentum nuchae*) are composed mostly of elastic fibers.

               (c) aponeuroses; although the layers may interweave, the composition is the same as tendons but they are broad and thin.

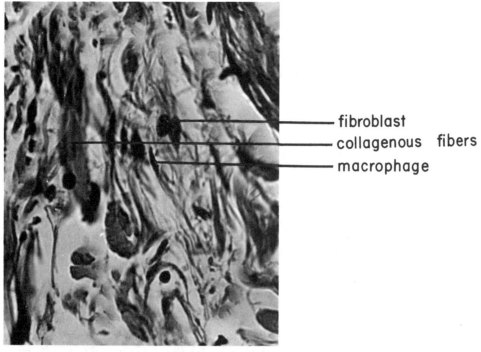

fibroblast
collagenous fibers
macrophage

Fibroelastic connective tissue

V.   BONE AND CARTILAGE

I.   SPECIALIZED CT

   A.   Cartilage and bone

      1.   Composed of cells, fibers, and ground substance whose matrix
           has a greater rigidity than CT Proper.

   B.   Cartilage

      1.   Hyaline (*nose, larynx, trachea, bronchi, articular surfaces of
           bones within joints, ear, and ventral ends of ribs*).
           a.   Cells
                (1)   chondrocytes (*to 40* μ) appear spherical with a
                      spherical nucleus centrally placed, one or more
                      nuclei, basophilic cytoplasm containing fat droplets
                      and glycogen, occur singly or as a cell nest.
           b.   Fibers
                (1)   collagen fibers form a fine network.
           c.   Ground substance
                (1)   stiff and gelatinous, about 70% water, includes
                      chondromucoid (*a glycoprotein*), chondroitin-sulfuric
                      acid, albuminoid, translucent, metachromatic with
                      toluidine blue, PAS positive, and basophilic. A
                      territorial matrix surrounds cell groups.
           d.   Perichondrium
                (1)   dense CT covering cartilage (except articular sur-
                      faces); fibroblasts, collagenous and elastic fibers;
                      inner cells can differentiate into chondrocytes.
           e.   Development
                (1)   mesenchymal cells become closely packed and collagen
                      fibers appear, matrix develops and the cells acquire
                      characteristics of chondrocytes.
           f.   Growth
                (1)   interstitial growth
                      (a)   young chondrocytes undergo mitosis and form cell
                            nests.
                (2)   appositional growth
                      (a)   fibroblasts from the inner layer of the peri-
                            chondrium, after mitosis, transform to chondro-
                            cytes, and lay down intercellular substance.
                            Injury may be repaired in this manner, also.

      2.   Elastic (*auricle, auditory tube, epiglottis, larynx-corniculate,
           cuniform, and arytenoid cartilages*).
           a.   Fundamentally, elastic cartilage is similar to the de-
                scription for hyaline cartilage. The major difference is
                the presence of many elastic fibers.

      3.   Fibrocartilage (*intervertebral discs and pubic symphysis*).

30

    a. Fibrocartilage is not considered as a modification of
        hyaline cartilage as is elastic cartilage; it never
        occurs alone, but merges with hyaline cartilage or dense
        fibrous CT: composed of bundles of dense collagenous
        fibers, interspaced with rows of chondrocytes; lacks a
        perichondrium.

C. Bone (*Osseous tissue*)

  1. Types
    a. Spongy (*cancellous*) - a meshwork of irregular bars or
        trabeculae of bone whose spaces are filled with bone
        marrow.
    b. Compact (*dense*) - appears solid, but contains the same
        histological elements as spongy bone.
    c. Long bones - compact bone forms the diaphysis which sur-
        rounds the bone marrow or medullary cavity. Each epi-
        physis consists of spongy bone covered by a thin shell of
        compact bone; medullary cavities are continuous.
    d. Flat bones - an inner and outer layer of compact bone
        encloses a middle layer of spongy bone (*diploë*).
    e. Irregular and short bones - spongy bone covered by a thin
        shell of compact bone.
  2. Structural elements
    a. Cells (*transform readily from one type to another*).
      (1) osteoblasts - usually found in a continuous layer
           associated with bone formation; large nucleus,
           prominent nucleolus, basophilic cytoplasm; active in
           bone formation.
      (2) osteocytes - considered a transformed osteoblast
           lying in a lacunae; fine cytoplasmic processes extend
           into the canaliculi radiating from lacunae.
      (3) osteoclasts - multinucleated cells usually at bone
           surface in Howship's lacunae; active in bone resorp-
           tion.
    b. Fibers
      (1) osteo-collagenous fibers in lamellae.
      (2) Sharpey's fibers are continuations of periosteal
           fibers (*dense fibrous CT*) consisting of collagenous
           or FECT bundles. Some elastic fibers are found ex-
           tending into the outer circumferential and intersti-
           tial lamellae, but not the Haversian systems; they
           are numerous where tendons and ligaments meet on bone.
    c. Matrix
      (1) ground substance is an acid mucopolysaccharide which
           acts as a cementing substance uniting fibers.
      (2) minerals present include calcium phosphate (*85%*),
           calcium carbonate (*10%*), and small amounts of calcium
           fluoride and magnesium fluoride. X-ray diffraction

                studies have shown that crystals of the minerals have
                a pattern of hydroxyapatites.
        d. Periosteum (*not on articular surfaces*)
            (1) outer dense fibrous CT layer with many vascular units,
                 nerves, and lymphatics.
            (2) inner osteogenic layer.
        e. Endosteum
            (1) formed of a delicate stratum of CT, containing osteo-
                 genic cells, which line marrow cavities.
        f. Marrow
            (1) red - consists of delicate reticular CT, osteogenic
                 cells, and hemopoietic cells.
            (2) yellow - mostly fat cells which have replaced other
                 marrow elements.
    3. Bone architecture
        a. Volkmann's Canals
            (1) canals from periosteal and endosteal surfaces con-
                 necting to Haversian canals thru which blood vessels,
                 lymphatics, and nerves pass.
        b. Haversian system (*osteone*)
            (1) Haversian canal - central and surrounded by concentric
                 lamellae.
            (2) canaliculi bordering the cavity of the canal bring all
            (3) lacunae (*space between lamellae containing osteocytes*)
                 of a system into continuity.
        c. Interstitial lamellae are matrix intervals between
            Haversian systems which are remnants of former H-S.
        d. Circumferential lamellae are periosteal and endosteal
            lamellae.
        e. Cement line - a thin layer of refractile modified matrix
            separating adjacent lamellae systems.
    4. Joints
        a. Bones are connected by articulations (*joints*).
        b. Synarthroses
            (1) immovable or slightly movable joints.
                (a) synostosis - bone connecting bone to bone.
                (b) synchondrosis - cartilage connecting bone to
                     bone.
                (c) syndesmosis - CT connecting bone to bone.
        c. Diarthroses
            (1) joints permit free movement of bones.
            (2) these joints contain a cavity.
            (3) walls of joint capsule.
                (a) fibrous layer (*external*) - dense CT which is
                     continuous with the periosteum.
                (b) synovial layer (*internal*) - cellular membrane
                     which may secrete synovial fluid into the joint
                     cavity.

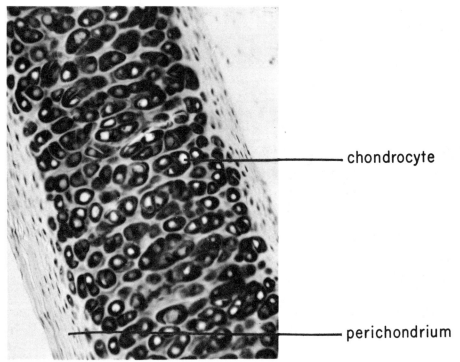

chondrocyte

perichondrium

Hyaline cartilage

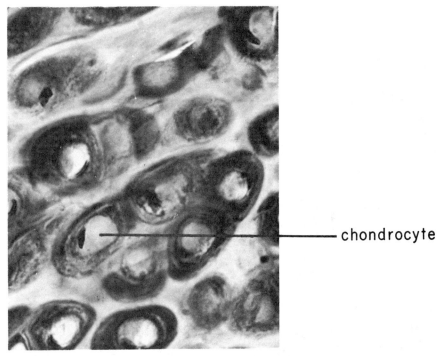

— chondrocyte

Elastic cartilage

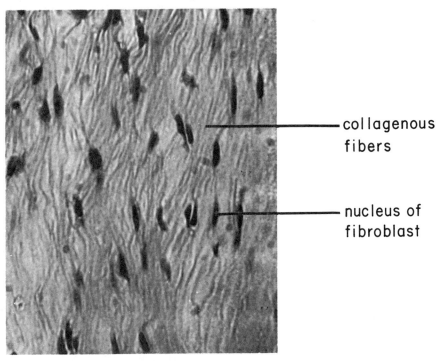

— collagenous
fibers

— nucleus of
fibroblast

Fibrocartilage

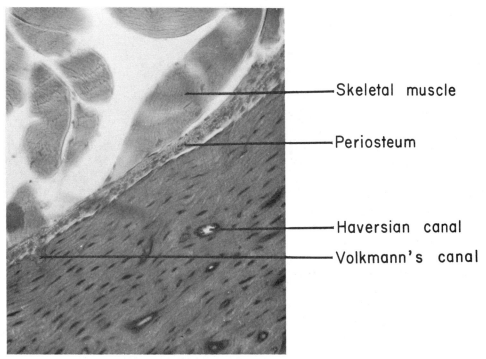

Compact Bone

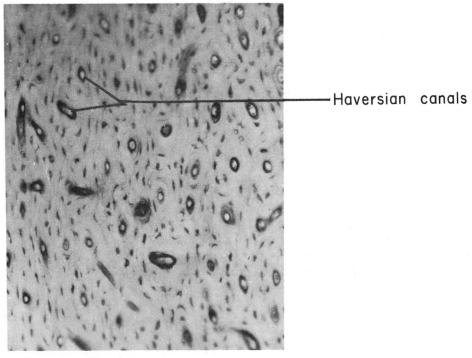

Compact Bone

VI. BONE: DEVELOPMENT; FRACTURE AND REPAIR

I. DEVELOPMENT

A. Embryological origin

1. Intramembranous
   a. Bone develops on or within a CT membrane.
   b. Removal of cartilage is not involved.
   c. Examples: flat bones of skull.
2. Intracartilaginous (*endochondral*)
   a. The fundamental process of bone deposition is the same in both types.
   b. Additionally, portions of cartilage are removed preparatory to bone deposition.

B. Intramembranous bone formation

1. Mesenchyme becomes highly vascularized and the active cells proliferate.
2. Mesenchyme cells enlarge and differentiate into osteoblasts.
3. Hyaline ground substance appears between osteoblasts which masks the collagenous fibers already present as well as those subsequently formed.
4. Osteoid is a matrix of intercellular substance and collagenous fibers not containing the inorganic constituent.
5. Lacunae and canaliculi form as osteoid surrounds osteoblasts.
6. Calcification of matrix occurs by deposition of bone salts intimately associated with collagenous fibers (*transformation may be the result of osteoblast activity*).
7. Plates and trabeculae are formed as the foci of bone formation which enclose spaces (*primary marrow cavities*).
8. These spaces are highly vascularized CT which become myeloid tissue.

C. Intracartilaginous bone formation

1. Ossification involves the replacement of a cartilage (*hyaline*) model by bone.
2. In long bones, ossification begins at the diaphyseal (*primary ossification*) center.
3. Cartilage cells proliferate, hypertrophy, and lacunae increase in size and number as the matrix becomes reduced between lacunae; these thin partitions calcify.
4. Concomitant with the intracartilaginous changes some of the inner cells of the perichondrium hypertrophy and become osteoblasts.
5. A bone ring or collar forms around the center of ossification.
6. The perichondrium differentiates into a periosteum, and vascular CT sprouts (*periosteal buds*) grow through the perforated bony collar from the periosteum into the changing cartilage matrix.

7. The vascular periosteal buds penetrate the thin-walled parti-
    tions between lacunae and form cavities called primary marrow
    spaces which contain blood vessels and embryonal CT cells.
    Some of these cells become osteoblasts aligned on calcified
    cartilage trabeculae which becomes enclosed by osteoid and then
    calcified bone. The trabeculae are a temporary supporting
    framework, and are subsequently resorbed as the marrow cavity
    enlarges.
8. The periosteal bone collar thickens, widens, and extends toward
    the epiphyses.
9. As ossification extends toward the ends of the cartilage, an
    orderly sequence of changes occurs so that several zones can
    be distinguished in the cartilage similar to that which took
    place in the development of the primary ossification center.
10. Zones of:
    a. Reserve (*quiescent*) cartilage
        (1) the primitive hyaline cartilage nearest the ends of
             the bone.
    b. Cell proliferation
        (1) a single cell in the reserve cartilage gives rise to
             a row of cells; each row arising is arranged parallel
             to the long axis of the cartilage model.
    c. Maturation
        (1) mitoses no longer occur and lacunae enlarge.
    d. Calcification
        (1) minerals deposit in the matrix surrounding the en-
             larged lacunae.
    e. Retrogression (*erosion*)
        (1) matrix between chondrocytes undergoes dissolution as
             do the cells, but the thicker matrix remains intact.
             Vascular primary marrow extends into the eroded
             spaces.
    f. Ossification
        (1) mesenchymal cells in the marrow tissue differentiate
             into osteoblasts which align on the calcified carti-
             lage plates and form bone.
    g. Resorption
        (1) resorption of bone occurs in diaphyseal center result-
             ing in an increase of size in the secondary marrow
             cavity. Simultaneously, ossification is advancing
             toward the ends of the cartilage.
        (2) as endochondral bone is resorbed centrally, the perio-
             steal collar thickens and extends toward the epiphyses.
11. Secondary ossification centers appear in each end of long bones.
    Ossification spreads in all directions except at two sites:
    a. Articular cartilage
    b. Epiphyseal plate (*disc*)
        (1) in the adult, when the epiphysis and diaphysis are
             united by bone, the epiphyseal line is formed and no
             increase in bone length is possible.

D. Fracture and repair

   1. After a fracture, torn vessels cause hemorrhage and clotting.
   2. A procallus results from fibroblasts and capillaries invading
       the clot and forming granulation tissue.
   3. The granulation tissue becomes dense fibrous tissue and trans-
       forms into a mass of cartilage which is the temporary callus
       that unites fractured bones.
   4. The temporary callus cartilage is replaced by spongy bone laid
       down by osteoblasts which develop from the periosteum and
       endosteum.
   5. The bony callus undergoes reorganization into compact bone.

VII. SPECIALIZED CONNECTIVE TISSUE - BLOOD

I. PERIPHERAL BLOOD

    A. Relation of blood to other CT.

        1. CT proper
           a. The intercellular ground substance is somewhat a jellied fibrous mass.
        2. Cartilage
           a. The intercellular ground substance masks the fibers in a rubbery consistency.
        3. Bone
           a. The intercellular ground substance is impregnated with calcium salts.
        4. Blood
           a. The intercellular ground substance is a liquid.

    B. Characteristics

        1. Red blood corpuscles
           a. Biconcave discs about 7.5 µ in D.
           b. RBC hematocrit is about 36 - 45.
           c. RBC count
               (1) males = 5.2×10^6/cmm.
               (2) females = 4.5×10^6/cmm.
        2. Blood volume
           a. About 7% of body weight.
        3. Types
           a. A = 41%
           b. O = 44%
           c. AB = 4%
           d. B = 11%
        4. Leukocytes
           a. Count = $5 - 9 \times 10^3$/cmm.
           b. All exhibit ameboid movement.
           c. Agranular.
               (1) lymphocytes
                   (a) 20 - 25% (*of total leukocytes*)
                   (b) seldom phagocytic
               (2) monocytes
                   (a) 3 - 8%
                   (b) sometimes phagocytic
           d. Granular
               (1) neutrophils
                   (a) 65 - 75%
                   (b) phagocytic
               (2) eosinophils
                   (a) 2 - 5%
                   (b) rarely phagocytic
               (3) basophils
                   (a) 0.5% or less
                   (b) rarely phagocytic

II. Hemopoiesis

    A. Theories

        1. Monophyletic
           a. Hemocytoblast
        2. Diphyletic
           a. Lymphoblast in lymphoid tissue
               (1) lymphocytes
               (2) monocytes
           b. Myeloblast in myeloid tissue
               (1) granular leucocytes
               (2) red blood cells
        3. Polyphyletic
           a. Lymphoblast........lymphocytes
           b. Monoblast.........monocytes
           c. Myeloblast........granular leucocytes and red blood cells

    B. Bone marrow

        1. Is 4 - 5% of body weight, and largest organ of the body.
        2. Yellow marrow consists mostly of fat cells.
        3. Red marrow is primarily in sternum, ribs, vertebrae, and
           proximal epiphyses of some long bones.
        4. Stroma of marrow
           a. Consists of reticular fibers, phagocytic reticular cells
              and some fat cells.
        5. Blood vessels of marrow
           a. Are large, tortuous sinusoids lined by flattened phago-
              cytic reticular cells (*macrophages which may detach and*
              become free). Although actually unknown, arteries may
              drain into arterioles-into capillaries-to sinusoids-to
              venules which exit at various sites of marrow. No lymph
              vessels have been demonstrated.
        6. Free cells
           a. All stages of cells in maturation of red and white cells
              are found in marrow.

    C. Sites

        1. Yolk sac........by third week.
        2. Liver..........by four--six weeks.
        3. Thymus.........by second month.
        4. Spleen.........by third month.
        5. Lymph nodes.....by third month.
        6. Bone marrow.....by third month.
           a. Marrow buds
           b. Marrow sprouts

HEMOPOIESIS

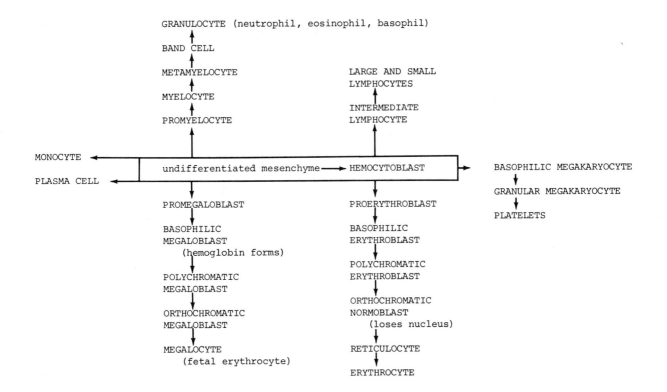

*Characteristics of the Various Blood Cells. (Stained by Wright's Method)

Cell	Size¹ microns	Cytoplasm				Nucleus			
		Amount	Stain²	Granules	Size	Shape	Stain²	Chromatin	Nucleolus
Reticulum cell	16-25 (long)	Narrow, long, branched	Light blue	None	Small	Round or oval	Light blue	Loosely reticulated	Distinct
Histiocyte	16-20	Wide zone Vacuoles	Light blue	None	Moderate	Kidney or bean	Light blue	Loosely reticulated	Distinct
Monoblast	14-20	Moderate	Deep blue	None	Large	Slightly indented, round or oval	Deep purple-blue	Fine chromatin structure	Indistinct but visible
Promonocyte	14-20	Moderate	Lighter blue	May appear	Large	Irregular	Purple-blue	Coarser	One or more nucleoli
Monocyte	14-20	Wide zone	Grayish-blue (slate color)	Dust-like, azurophilic or red Oxidase positive	Moderate	Indented, lobulated; occasionally round or oval	Light purple-blue	Compact, coarse, spongy, reticulated	Absent
Myeloblast	12-20	Narrow to moderate	Bright sky blue	Fine granules Oxidase positive	Large	Round or oval	Light purple-blue	Finely reticulated and sieve-like	Indistinct but visible Usually multiple
Progranulocyte	9-20	Moderate	Less deeply blue	Deeply azurophilic, coarse granules may cover nuclear chromatin	Large	Oval or kidney	Light purple-blue	More coarse than blast cell	Distinct if present
Myelocyte	9-18	Moderate	Light violet	Granules start differentiating	Large	Round or oval	Dark purple-blue	Net form, more compact	Rare (indistinct)
Metamyelocyte	9-16	Wide zone	Lilac-blue	Neut.: fine, purple Oxy.: coarse, red Baso.: coarse, blue-black	Moderate	Indented, bean or kidney shaped	Purple	Fine strands, more compact	None
Band cell	9-16	Wide zone	Neut.: lilac Oxy.: light blue Baso.: light blue	Neut.: lilac Oxy.: red Baso.: blue-black	Moderate	Curved or coiled band	Purple	More compact	None

Segmented granulocytes (a) Neutrophil (b) Eosinophil (c) Basophil	9-12	Wide zone	(a) Lilac or salmon pink (b) and (c) faint sky blue	(a) Lilac dust (b) Red, distinct (c) Blue-black, distinct	Moderate	Segmented: (a) 3-5 seg. (b) 2 seg. (c) 2 seg.	(a) Dense purple; (b) and (c) less dense	Coarse strands, still more compact	None
Lymphoblast	15-20	Abundant	Less blue than myeloblast	Oxidase negative Azure granules may be present	Large	Round or oval	Light purple-blue	Fine chromatin structure	Distinct Usually single
Prolymphocyte	12-15 or larger	Abundant	Light blue	Azurophilic may be present More coarse than in monocyte	Large	Round or oval	Deep purple-blue	Coarse trabeculae rather than threads	Usually present
Lymphocyte	6-10	Narrow rim	Robin's egg blue	None	Moderate	Round or slightly indented	Deep purple-blue	Compact heavy blocks	May be present
Proplasmacyte	15-20	Wide zone Vacuoles	Deep blue	Occasionally a few azurophilic granules	Large	Round or oval	Deep purple-red	Trabeculated	Present
Plasmacyte	8-15	Abundant Vacuoles	Deep blue	Occasionally a few azurophilic granules	Large	Round, eccentric	Deep reddish-blue	Large coarse clumps	Absent
Pronormoblast	15-20	Abundant	Deep blue	None	Large	Round or oval	Light purple-blue	Dense, net; coarser than the myeloblast	Present
Basophilic Normoblast	10-12	Wide zone	Navy blue	None	Large	Round	Purple-blue	More compact	Absent
Normoblast (Polychromatophilic to Acidophilic)	6-11	Abundant	Faint purple to red or buff	None	Young: large Old: small	Round	Deep purple	Shrunken, compact and pyknotic	Absent
Erythrocyte	6-10	Total	Orange or buff	None	None				
Megakaryoblast	16-25	Abundant	Light blue	None	Large	Lobulated	Dark purple-blue	Finely reticulated	Distinct
Megakaryocyte	12-75	Abundant	Light purple-blue	Azurophilic	Moderate	Lobulated	Dark purple-blue	More compact	None
Thrombocyte	2-4	Total	Pale blue	Azurophilic	None				

1 Size of cell varies with thickness of film.

2 The exact color depends upon the staining technic

*From Levinson, S. A. and MacFate, R. P. Clinical Laboratory Diagnosis. Table 15-4, pp. 760-761. Lea & Febiger, Philadelphia, 1969.

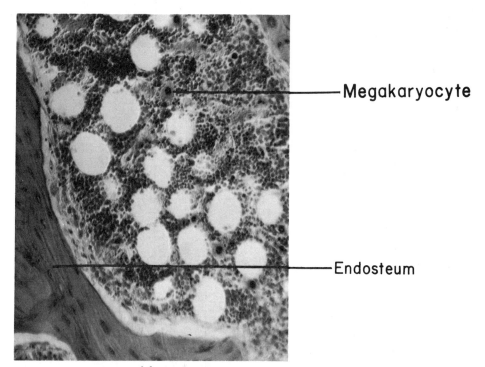

Megakaryocyte

Endosteum

Bone Marrow

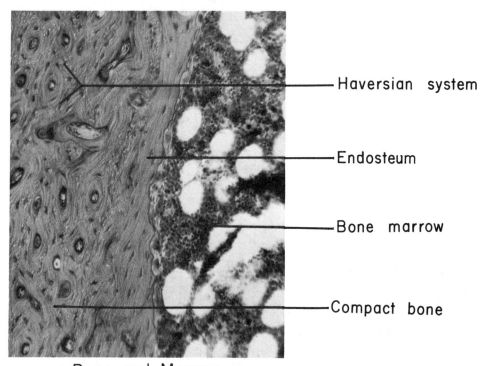

Haversian system

Endosteum

Bone marrow

Compact bone

Bone and Marrow

VIII. MUSCLE TISSUE

I. SMOOTH MUSCLE

A. General characteristics

1. Cells develop from embryonic mesenchyme, and may increase in size (*hypertrophy*) and perhaps by number (*hyperplasia*).
2. Tissue is found scattered singly or in bundles (*dermis*), intimately associated with CT, and in sheets (*as circular and longitudinal in the intestine*).
3. The tissue is found in the wall of the viscera supplying it with either movement or tonus (*sustained contraction*).
4. Examples - wall of alimentary canal from middle of esophagus to anus, gall bladder and hepatic ducts, wall of trachea and bronchial tree, ureter, urinary bladder, urethra, corpora cavernosa, testes and ducts, prostate gland, Cowper's glands, broad ligament, oviduct, uterus, vagina, blood vessels, spleen, large lymph vessels, arrectores pilorum, iris and ciliary body.

B. Cells (*often called fibers*)

1. Fusiform shape, abundant cytoplasm, and the nucleus lies in the thick central portion.
2. Length varies from 15 to 200 μ; diameter from 3 to 8 μ. In the pregnant uterus the length may reach 500 μ.
3. The nucleus conforms to cell shape, contains one or more nucleoli, has a fine chromatin network, and does not stain darkly.
4. The cytoplasm (*sarcoplasm*) is acidophilic, contains the usual organelles, and also longitudinally aligned myofibrils (*specialized structures for possible contraction*).
5. Myofibrils are more easily seen in fresh preparations (*macerated in 10% hydrochloric acid*). Apparently they represent aggregates of the EM myofilaments. It is known that the myofilaments contain actin and myosin although the EM has not revealed two types of filaments (*as it has for skeletal muscle*).
6. EM studies of the cytoplasmic membrane indicate a unit membrane; a fusion of the outer layers of adjacent cells has been termed a "nexus" indicating a more intimate cell union than desmosomes. There are nerve endings about some cells.
7. Myo-epithelial cells are cells in relation to some glands (*salivary, sweat, and lacrimal*) which have developed from ectoderm, but resemble smooth muscle cells in appearance.

II. SKELETAL MUSCLE

A. General characteristics

1. The supporting CT elements of the muscle are continuous with the CT structure to which it is attached such as tendon, aponeurosis, periosteum, dermis or other dense CT structure; the elements are

45

a. Epimysium
   (1) FECT sheath surrounding an entire muscle.
b. Perimysium
   (1) FECT which divides a muscle into different bundles
       (*fasciculi*).
c. Endomysium
   (1) a delicate network of reticular fibers surrounding
       each muscle cell; capillaries are carried in the
       fibrous network.
2. Muscles (*individual cells*) increase in size with exercise.
3. Skeletal muscles are products of myotomes and lateral plate
   mesoderm.

B. Cells (*often called fibers*)

1. Each cell is a long, cylindrical fiber tapering at each end;
   its length varies from 1 to 40 mm. or longer, and its diameter
   varies from 10 to 100 μ.
2. The cell is multinucleate; nuclei occur about 35 per mm. length,
   and locate peripherally.
3. Muscle cells exhibit "cross striations" along their course -
   hence they are also termed striated muscle fibers.
4. A muscle cell contains longitudinal myofibrils separated from
   each other by sarcoplasm (*muscle cytoplasm*) in which the usual
   cell organelles appear.
5. A cell is bounded by a sarcolemma. It consists of the cytoplasmic membrane covered by a fine basement membrane and a few
   unit fibers of FECT. Myofibrils are connected to the sarcolemma which in turn is connected to the endomysium. Numerous
   mitochondria are present between myofibrils.

C. Elements of contraction

1. A myofibril (*2-3* μ *D*) shows alternate dark A bands (*A for
   anisotropic*) and light I bands (*I for isotropic*). Each I band
   is bisected by a thin dark disc called the Z line (*Z for
   Zwischenscheibe = intermediate disc*). A pale thin H band bi-
   sects the A band, and a fine, dark M band lies in the H band.
   The N band lies in the I band between the Z and A bands.
2. A portion of one myofibril between two Z discs is called a
   sarcomere which is 2-3 μ long.
3. Although the myofibrils are the components of the fiber which
   contract, the contractile unit is the sarcomere.
4. In a cross-section of a muscle cell, bundles of myofibrils are
   seen as dots and separated by clear sarcoplasm - fields of
   Cohnheim.
5. Myofibrils contain myofilaments.
6. The filaments do not extend the whole length of the sarcomere,
   and there are two different kinds - fine (*actin*) and coarse
   (*myosin*) filaments.

7. Fine filaments attach to Z discs and extend toward the middle where they terminate in free ends; the gaps between the free ends form the H band.

8. The spinous course filaments are confined to the A band where they interdigitate with the smooth fine filaments.

9. In the "sliding theory of contraction", the A band and I band diminish.

D. Impulse-transmission correlation

1. A motor unit is a single nerve fiber (*axon*) extending from a terminal branch of a peripheral nerve to a variable number of striated muscle cells.

2. The sheath of Schwann and the myelin sheath (*described under "Nerve Tissue"*) are lost from the axon as it approaches the muscle cell. The endoneurium appears to become continuous with the endomysium.

3. Contact between axon and sarcoplasm is made at the sole plasm. The axon shows a terminal dilation containing many small synaptic (*cytoplasmic*) vesicles which may contain acetylcholine. The junction is termed a motor end plate or myoneural junction.

4. Myofibrils are surrounded by sarcoplasmic (*endplasmic*) reticulum. The reticulum is composed of
   a. Centrotubules which encircle the myofibril at the Z disk and each has its beginning as a funnel-like opening (*invagination*) of the sarcolemma. The centrotubule is continuous with
   b. Distended sacs lying on either side of the centrotubule surrounding each sarcomere over each of its I bands, and
   c. Longitudinal tubules which lie over the A band, and connect the sacs with the flat
   d. H zone sacs

5. It is possible, then, to conceive that an impulse reaching the myoneural junction could cause a wave of depolarization to spread deep into a muscle cell via the tubular system so as to effect a sudden muscle contraction in every sarcomere.

III. CARDIAC MUSCLE

A. General characteristics

1. The myocardium of the heart is composed of striated muscle cells which are separated into bundles by CT. Vessels and nerves are located within the CT. The bundles course in different directions, but the cells are roughly parallel.

2. Cardiac muscle cells do not form a syncytium.

3. The myocardium is derived from the splanchnic mesoderm.

B. Cells

1. Nuclei tend to be disposed centrally in the cells and are
    usually ovoid in shape.
2. Sarcoplasm extends between myofibrils and contains numerous
    mitochondria.
3. Myofibrils are similar to those in skeletal muscle cells, and
    show the same bands, but not as distinct. Contraction of the
    myofilaments is thought to be the same as in skeletal muscle.
4. Sarcolemma consists of elements similar to those of skeletal
    muscle cells.
5. Intercalated discs are the sites of end to end attachments of
    cardiac muscle cells. They cross cells at Z lines. The thin
    actin filaments from terminal sarcomeres attach to the cyto-
    plasmic membranes.
6. Pigment of a brownish tinge is prominent with age, and is
    found in sarcoplasm near nuclei.
7. Purkinje fibers are specialized cardiac muscle cells which
    form a part of the impulse conduction system and are found
    beneath the endocardium. They have centrally disposed nuclei,
    cross striations, and intercalated disks. The myofibrils in a
    cell tend to locate peripherally, and glycogen accumulates in
    the central core.

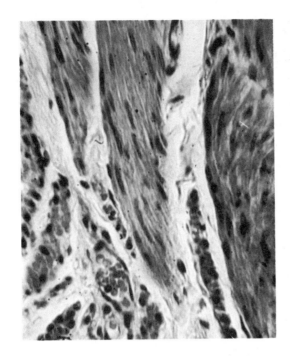

Smooth Muscle

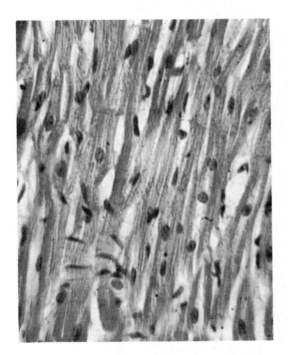

Cardiac Muscle

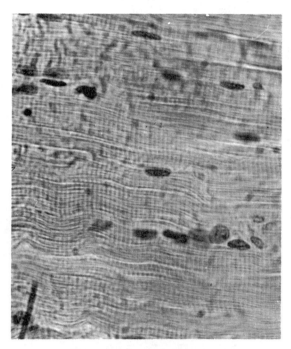

Skeletal   muscle

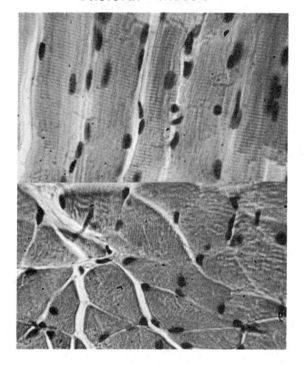

IX. NERVE TISSUE

I. MORPHOGENESIS OF NERVE TISSUE

A. Neural tube

1. After the formation of endoderm, mesoderm, and ectoderm in the
    embryo, the ectoderm in the mid-line thickens and forms the
    neural plate. A neural groove appears in the plate, and the
    elevations of either side become the neural folds. Some
    ectoderm bulges laterally from the folds forming the neural
    crests as the neural fold edges come together and fuse in the
    mid-line. The fusion forms the neural tube. The neuro-
    ectodermal cells of the neural tube later develop into the CNS
    while those from the neural crests give rise to the PNS.
    a. The inner layer (*ependymal layer*) of the neural tube dif-
        ferentiates into the ependyma,
    b. The middle layer (*mantle layer*) into the gray matter, and
        the
    c. Outer layer (*marginal layer*) into the white matter. Al-
        though in the cortex of the cerebral and cerebellar hemi-
        spheres neuroblasts from the middle layer migrate through
        the outer layer to locate peripherally.

B. Neural divisions

1. Spinal cord
    a. The lateral walls of the neural tube thicken and the cells
        proliferate to form
        (1) roof plate (*dorsal*)
        (2) floor plate (*ventral*)
        (3) sulcus limitans - depression in the cavity of the
             neural tube (*central canal*) between dorsal and
             ventral thickenings of the lateral walls.
        (4) alar plates - dorsal thickenings
        (5) basal plates - ventral thickenings
        (6) dorsal septum - fusion of dorsal lumen
        (7) central canal - neural tube lumen
2. Primary vesicles
    a. The anterior end of the neural tube forms three vesicles
        and two constrictions.
        (1) hindbrain (*rhombencephalon*)
             (a) hindpart (*myelencephalon*) - medulla oblongata.
             (b) constriction - pontine flexure.
             (c) forepart (*metencephalon*) - pons from the floor
                  and cerebellum from lateral swellings.
             (d) lumen - fourth ventricle.
             (e) vellum - thin roof plate, fourth ventricle.
        (2) midbrain (*mesencephalon*)
             (a) lumen-aqueduct.
        (3) constriction - cephalic flexure.

51

        (4)   forebrain (*prosencephalon*)
           (a) hindpart (*diencephalon*) - thalamus, hypothalamus, subthalamus, third ventricle
           (b) forepart (*telencephalon*) - cerebral hemispheres, and first and second ventricles

C. Histogenesis of CNS

  1. Cells
    a. Neuroepithelial cells of the inner germinal layer are pushed into the middle tube layer that differentiate into
      (1) neuroblasts which become
        (a) neurons, and
      (2) free spongioblasts which become either
        (a) astroblasts which become
          (1) protoplasmic astrocytes of gray matter, or
          (2) fibrous astrocytes of white matter.
    b. Germinal cells of the inner layer of the neural tube remain and differentiate into
      (1) ependymal spongioblasts which become
      (2) ependymal cells lining the central canal of the cord and the brain ventricles.
    c. Most of the axons in the outer layer become covered with myelin to give the white matter appearance.
    d. Neurons
      (1) multipolar when possessing one axon and two or more dendrites; cell body (*perikaryon*) contains nucleus which is large, spherical and vesicular with a nucleolus; the usual cytoplasmic organelles, neurofibrils and neurofilaments; the two pigments, lipochrome and melanin, and Nissl bodies which are aggregations of rough-surfaced flattened endoplasmic reticulum.
    e. Neuroglia
      (1) astrocytes with large and round nuclei
        (a) fibrous (*white matter*)
        (b) protoplasmic (*gray matter*)
      (2) oligodendroglia with small round nuclei
      (3) microglia (*derived from mesoderm*) with elongated and narrow nuclei

II. NERVOUS SYSTEM

A. Central nervous system

  1. Brain
  2. Spinal cord

B. Peripheral nervous system

    1. Nerves
    2. Ganglia
    3. Nerve endings

C. Autonomic nervous system

    1. Sympathetic division (*thoraco-lumbar*)
    2. Parasympathetic division (*cranio-sacral*)

D. Reflex arc

E. Synapse

F. Components of nervous system

    1. Neurons
    2. Interstitial tissue
        a. Neuroglia of CNS
        b. Neurolemma of peripheral nerve fibers
        c. Satellite cells of cerebrospinal and sympathetic ganglia
    3. Connective tissue
        a. Meninges of CNS
        b. Sheaths of peripheral nerves

III. THE MENINGES

  A. CT membranes

    1. Pia mater
        a. Innermost meninx covering the brain and spinal cord
        b. Consists of delicate FECT covered by squamous cells
           similar to those of mesothelial membranes.
        c. It contains fibroblasts, macrophages, and many blood
           vessels which penetrate the brain.
    2. Arachnoid
        a. Middle meninx of delicate FECT is connected to the pia
           mater by a network of trabeculae (*and often is termed*
           pia-arachnoid or leptomeninx).
        b. The membrane and trabeculae are covered by squamous cells
           similar to those of the pia.
        c. This membrane does not extend into the sulci as does the
           pia.
        d. Cerebrospinal fluid fills the pia-arachnoid spaces
           (*cisternae*).
    3. Dura mater
        a. Outermost meninx of dense FECT.
        b. Subdural space separates dura from arachnoid.
        c. In the cranium the dura is fused with the internal perio-
           steum, but not in the spinal cord.

IV. CEREBROSPINAL FLUID

    A. Formation

        1. It occupies the brain ventricles, central canal of the spinal
           cord, the subarachnoid and perivascular spaces; its quantity
           may be as much as 150 ml.
        2. Telae choroideae is composed of two membranes.
           a. The inner membrane is the ependymal layer.
           b. The outer membrane is the pia mater.
           c. Blood vessels lie between the two membranes at the level
              of the choroid plexus.
           d. The telae forms the roofs of the first and second ventricles.
        3. The choroid plexuses project into the ventricles from the
           telae choroideae as complex folds containing networks of ves-
           sels derived from those of the pia.
        4. Evidence indicates that the cerebrospinal fluid is formed by
           the activity of cuboidal epithelial cells of the ependymal
           layer lining the choroid plexus and telae as well as filtration
           fluid from the capillaries in the plexuses.

    B. Circulation and absorption

        1. The fluid passes into the ventricles and then into the sub-
           achnoid spaces via foramen of Magendie and the two foramina
           of Luschka; these three openings are in the roof of the fourth
           ventricle.
        2. The fluid apparently filters through the arachnoid villi to
           drain into the cerebral venous sinuses.

V. SPINAL CORD, CEREBELLAR AND CEREBRAL CORTEX

    A. Spinal cord

        1. Gray matter
           a. Is arranged in the shape of the letter H with the points
               forming the anterior and posterior horns.
           b. Multipolar neuron cell bodies, portions of dendrites and
               some myelinated and non-myelinated axonic fibers held to-
               gether by neuroglia cells.
        2. White matter
           a. Is composed of myelinated and non-myelinated fibers, neu-
               roglia, blood vessels, and inward extensions of the pia
               mater.

    B. Cerebellar cortex

        1. Cerebellum
           a. It is connected to the brain by three peduncles.

    b. It consists of two hemispheres (*lateral lobes*) interconnected by the vermis (*medium lobe*).

    c. Each lobe has fissures demarking lobules whose surfaces have folds (*folia or laminae*) parallel to the fissures. The folds have secondary and tertiary folia giving an appearance in sagittal sections called the arbor vitae.

    d. A cortex forms the surface of gray matter which envelops white matter; it has three layers
        (1) the outer (*molecular or plexiform*) layer of stellate cells
        (2) the inner (*granular or nuclear*) layer, and
        (3) the Purkinje cells which are large and pear-shaped that form a single row between the outer and inner layers.

C. Cerebral cortex

    1. Cerebrum
        a. Is composed of two hemispheres with convolutions and fissures.
        b. The cortex is the external layer of gray matter containing fibers, neuroglia, blood vessels, and an estimated 14×10^9 cell bodies of neurons. Six layers may be exhibited:
            (1) molecular layer
            (2) outer granular layer
            (3) outer pyramidal cell layer
            (4) inner granular layer
            (5) inner pyramidal layer
            (6) multiform layer

VI. PERIPHERAL NERVOUS SYSTEM

A. Nerves

    1. Spinal nerves are fibers connected with the spinal cord.
        a. Somatic efferent fibers (*motor to skeletal muscles*)
        b. Visceral efferent fibers (*motor to smooth muscles*)
        c. Somatic afferent fibers (*sensory from skin*)
        d. Visceral afferent fibers (*sensory from viscera*)
    2. Cranial nerves are fibers connected with the brain.
        a. Some are efferent, some are afferent, and others contain both efferent and afferent fibers.
    3. Structure
        a. Epineurium is a CT sheath of FECT with fibroblasts and macrophages enclosing the nerve.
        b. Perineurium is the fine CT epineurium extension surrounding the nerve fasciculi.
        c. Endoneurium is the perineurium extension of delicate CT surrounding each nerve fiber.
        d. Myelin sheath

       e. Neurolemma (*sheath of Schwann*) contain Schwann cells
          which form myelin.
       f. Node of Ranvier
       g. Incisures of Schmidt-Lantermann
  4. Fibers of Remak
       a. Non-myelinated nerve fibers in the PNS.

B. Ganglia

  1. An aggregate of nerve cell bodies outside the CNS; in the CNS
      the aggregation is generally called a nucleus.
      a. Types
          (1) craniospinal - sensory ganglia
          (2) autonomic - visceral, motor ganglia
  2. General characteristics
      a. Size varies from few to perhaps 5×10^3 cell bodies.
      b. A CT capsule is continuous with the epineurium and peri-
          neurium surrounding each ganglion; it contains blood ves-
          sels.
      c. Fibers are present.
      d. Capsule (*or satellite*) cells form a single layer around
          each ganglion cell.
  3. Spinal ganglia are located on the posterior roots of spinal
      nerves.
  4. Cranial ganglia are located on some cranial nerves.
  5. The autonomic nervous system is constituted by efferent
      neurons which innervate smooth and caridac muscles, and glands
      of the body.
      a. Autonomic ganglia are located
          (1) on the sympathetic chain, and
          (2) as four ganglia (*ciliary, spheno-palatine, otic, and
              submandibular* (*and sublingual*) which are related to
              the cranial parasympathetic system, and
          (3) in the walls of the organs supplied by the parasym-
              pathetic system.

C. Nerve endings

  1. Somatic efferent fibers terminate in motor end plates.
  2. Visceral efferent fibers form plexuses around muscle bundles.
      Fine fibers from the plexuses end as enlarged nodules on or
      within the muscle cells; in glands, the fibers terminate as
      free endings on the gland cells.
  3. Receptors
      a. Receive stimuli, and contain the terminations of peri-
          pheral afferent fibers.
      b. Somaesthetic
      c. Organs of special senses
      d. Exteroceptors
      e. Proprioceptors
      f. Enteroceptors

4. Afferent fibers
    a. Free or non-encapsulated endings in epithelia, CT, muscle,
        and serous membranes.
        (1) tactile corpuscle of Merkel (*in skin*)
    b. Encapsulated endings
        (1) end bulbs of Krause in conjunctival CT
        (2) tactile corpuscles of Meissner in fingertips, soles,
             and palms lying in CT dermal papillae
        (3) Pacinian corpuscle (*corpuscle of Vater-Pacini*) in
             deep subcutaneous CT of hand and foot, pancreas,
             mammary gland, penis, clitoris, parietal peritoneum,
             and mesentery.
        (4) muscle spindles or neuromuscular bundles in skeletal
             muscle
5. An axon may end in an aborization called telodendria; the end-
    point terminus is an expansion called an end bulb in which
    numerous mitochondria and synaptic vessels (*with acetylcholine*)
    are located.
6. Synapse
    a. The synapse is the point of close approximation (*area
        about 200 A wide*) between two neurons where an impulse is
        transmitted from one to another.
7. Reflex arc
    a. Is the intergrative unit of the whole nervous system. The
        impulse pathway can be illustrated with a generalized
        three-neuron reflex arc.
        (1) in a receptor site, a dendrite of a sensory (*afferent
             neuron*), whose cell body lies in a posterior root
             ganglion, receives a stimulus which is transmitted
             from the ganglion via the axon into the spinal cord
             where it synapses with a
        (2) connector (*association, or internuncial*) neuron in
             the gray matter. At this point there are potentially
             numerous pathways established in the CNS. Synapse
             occurs with a
        (3) motor (*efferent*) neuron in the anterior horn of gray
             matter whose axon conducts the impulse in a peripheral
             nerve to a skeletal muscle in an effector site.

58

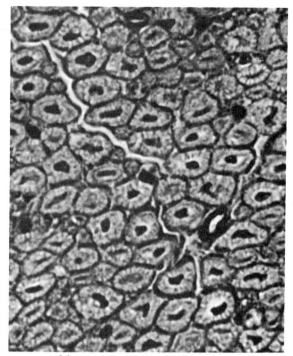

Nerve, cross-section

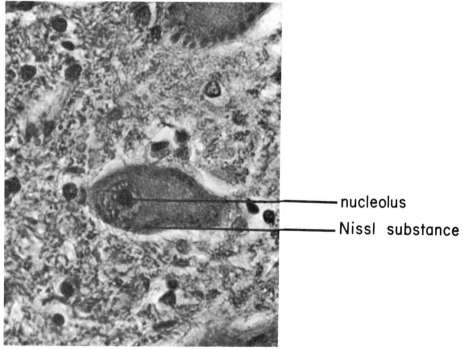

nucleolus

Nissl substance

Nerve cell body

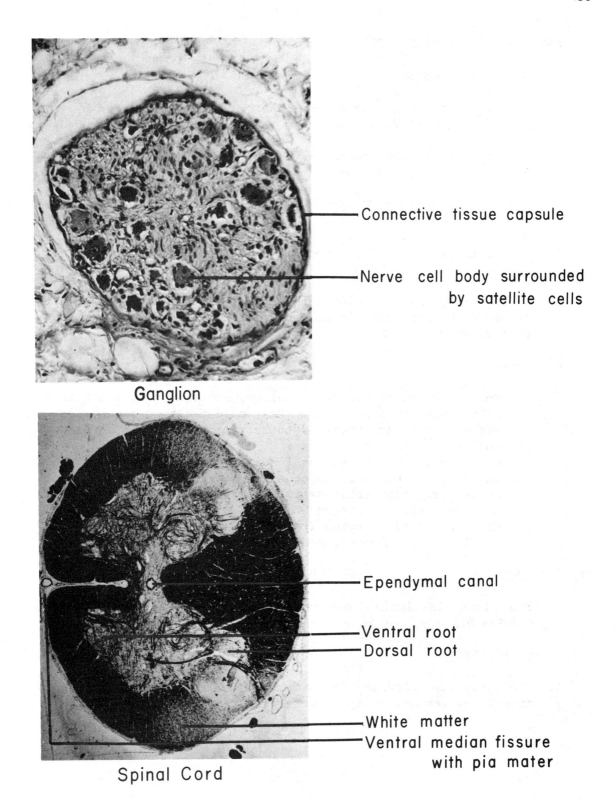

Connective tissue capsule

Nerve cell body surrounded by satellite cells

Ganglion

Ependymal canal

Ventral root
Dorsal root

White matter
Ventral median fissure with pia mater

Spinal Cord

X.   THE CIRCULATORY SYSTEM

I.   CAPILLARIES (*AVERAGE* = *8*μ)

   A.   Endothelial cells

      1.   These simple squamous tube-like cells are surrounded by thin
           and delicate collagenous and reticular fibers in a ground sub-
           stance.
      2.   Connect arterioles and venules.
      3.   Lie on a basement membrane.

   B.   Pericapillary cells: Rouget cells which are probably macrophages
        or undifferentiated mesenchymal cells.

   C.   Mesh density: generally proportional to metabolic intensity of
        tissue.

   D.   Permeability (*rate*): related to rate of blood flow, hydrostatic
        pressure, colloid osmotic pressure (*within and without*), tissue
        turgor, gravity, etc.

   E.   Types

      1.   Those with continuous endothelium, continuous basement mem-
           brane, sometimes with pericytes, no detectable cement sub-
           stance, no pores but pinocytotic vesicles on both surfaces,
           and in
           a.   Cardiac muscle, skeletal muscle, CT, and lung.
      2.   Those with continuous endothelium, continuous basement mem-
           brane, few pinocytotic vesicles, glial end-feet on external
           surface mostly in CNS and retina.
      3.   Fenestrated capillaries (*pores*)
           a.   Intestinal mucosa, and kidney glomerulus.

II.   SINUSOIDS

   A.   Wide, irregular lumina sometimes lined by cells of RES
        (*review histology of bone marrow, lymph nodes, and liver*).

III.   RETE MIRABILE

   A.   Capillary-like plexus (*sinusoid*) inserted in the course of an
        arteriole, venule, or lymph vessel (not in man).

IV. STRUCTURAL PLAN OF BLOOD VESSELS

   A. General differences between artery and vein

      1. Luminal bore to wall thickness
      2. Regularity of lumen
      3. Differentiation of layers within the wall

   B. Tunica intima

      1. Endothelium (*simple squamous epithelium*)
      2. Subendothelial fibro-elastic connective tissue
      3. Internal elastic membrane

   C. Tunica media

      1. Smooth muscle
      2. Elastic fibers
      3. Fenestrated plates

   D. Tunica adventitia

      1. External elastic membrane
      2. FECT grades off into loose supporting CT

   E. Vasa vasorum

      1. These are nutrient vessels to
          a. arteries - mostly the adventitia.
          b. veins - may extend thru the media.

   F. Lymphatics

      1. In wall of the larger blood vessels

   G. Nerves

      1. Unmyelinated (*vasomotor*) fibers in adventitia terminating on
          smooth muscle of media.
      2. Myelinated (*sensory*) fibers in adventitia which may reach
          intima.

V. SMALL ARTERIES - ARTERIOLES (*20 TO 500* μ)

   A. Intima: endothelium, basement membrane, minimal FECT internal
       elastic membrane.

   B. Media: smooth muscle (*quantity is roughly proportional to the
       caliber of the vessel*), FECT.

C. Adventitia: FECT, and no definite external elastic membrane.

VI. MEDIUM ARTERIES (*0.5 MM TO 1 CM*)

A. These are most of the named arteries in the body.

B. Intima: endothelium, FECT, and prominent internal elastic membrane which appears in cross-section as scalloped bundles of elastic fibers.

C. Media: smooth muscle with FECT; reticular fibers; separate internal and external elastic membranes; elastic is attached to basement membrane of muscle cells suggesting contractility relationship.

D. Adventitia: as thick or thicker than media with loose FECT.

VII. LARGE ARTERIES (*LARGER THAN 1 CM. – E.G., AORTA, SUBCLAVIAN AND CAROTID*)

A. Intima: polygonal endothelial cells, FECT with scattered bundles of smooth muscle, and internal elastic membrane not well-defined.

B. Media: abundant fenestrated, elastic bands of tissue interspersed with FECT and smooth muscle cells attached to elastic framework.

C. Adventitia: thin; FECT, external elastic membrane not well-defined.

VIII. SPECIAL ARTERIES

A. Cerebral and dural arteries: exceedingly thin walls and differ from other arteries in

1. Well-developed internal elastic membrane.
2. Little elastic tissue between smooth muscle cells in media.
3. Striking decrease of elastic fibers in adventitia.

B. Others

1. Celiac, femoral, radial are large-sized arteries which have walls like medium arteries.
2. Arteries of lower extremity have media thicker than similar-sized arteries elsewhere.
3. Umbilical arteries have an intima of only endothelial cells, a media of two well-defined smooth muscle layers, no internal or external elastic membranes, but elastic fibers present.
4. Pulmonary arteries, thin walls being reduced in smooth muscle and elastic fibers.
5. Uterine and ovarian arteries vary in structure during pregnancy and menstrual cycle.

C. Age change

   1. Architectural changes in many arteries begin during and after
       second decade of life, e.g., loss of elasticity (*distensibil-
       ity*) of large arteries.

IX. SMALL VEINS - VENULES (*20 µ TO 1 MM*)

   A. Intima: endothelium and collagenous fibers.

   B. Media: few smooth cells appear in larger vessels of this caliber,
       but not well defined.

   C. Adventitia: FECT appears.

X. MEDIUM VEINS (*1 MM TO 1 CM*)

   A. Intima: endothelium and FECT.

   B. Media: smooth muscle and collagen fibers not well developed; ill-
       defined internal elastic membrane.

   C. Adventitia: a few smooth cells and FECT.

XI. LARGE VEINS (*LARGER THAN 1 CM.; EXAMPLE, INFERIOR VENA CAVA*)

   A. Intima: endothelium and FECT.

   B. Media: small amount of smooth muscle cells and collagen fibers.

   C. Adventitia: much larger than media; FECT and longitudinal smooth
       muscle.

XII. SPECIAL VEINS

   A. Lacking smooth muscle; cavernous veins of erectile tissue, sub-
       capillary veins of skin, dural sinuses, most of pia and cerebral
       veins, retina, and some of placenta.

XIII. VALVES

   A. Projection of intima comprised of endothelium, elastic tissue, and
       a few smooth muscle cells.

XIV. ARTERIOVENOUS ANASTOMOSES

   A. Direct connection of arteriole to venule.

B. Arterial cushions: thickening of intima which acts like a valve on
    contraction of vessels such as umbilical, thyroid, bronchial,
    renal and prostatic vessels.

C. Carotid bodies: lie close to bifurcation of common carotid: com-
    posed of epitheloid cells resting against endothelium of sinusoidal
    capillaries. Nerve fibers enter and end on epitheloid cells. The
    bodies are considered as chemoreceptors for internal common carotid
    and are oxygen tension sensitive.

D. Aortic body: consists of epitheloid cells from aortic arch to base
    of heart; less circumscribed than the carotid body, but function-
    ally similar.

E. Coccygeal body: a small round mass of arteriovenous anastomoses
    consisting of a thick epitheloid layer of cells which lie close to
    the endothelium of tortuous blood vessels whose function is un-
    known.

XV. HEART

A. Endocardium

    1. Inner wall is homologous to the tunica intima of blood ves-
        sels.
    2. Endothelium and basement membrane
    3. Subendothelial layer of collagenous fibers
    4. FECT layer with a few smooth muscle cells
    5. Subendocardial layer of loose CT which binds the endocardium
        to myocardium; may contain blood vessels; nerves; fat cells;
        lymph vessels; and Purkinje fibers.

B. Myocardium

    1. Middle wall corresponding to tunica media.
    2. Composed of cardiac muscle arranged in sheets with intercellu-
        lar FECT.

C. Epicardium (*visceral pericardium*)

    1. Outer wall is homologous to the tunica adventitia.
    2. FECT is covered with mesothelium.
    3. An ill-defined subepicardial layer of loose CT attaches it to
        the myocardium.

D. Cardiac skeleton

    1. Dense fibrous CT on which cardiac muscle inserts.
    2. Composed of fibrous rings and fibrous trigones. Amorphous
        matrix may contain chondroitin sulfate and take basophilic
        stain.

E. Cardiac valves

    1. A reduplication of endocardium.
    2. Each bicuspid and tricuspid valve has a core of dense FECT
        whose base is continous with a fibrous ring. A few smooth
        muscle cells are present. Each valve connects to a papillary
        muscle by dense fibrous cords (*chordae tendinae*).
    3. Semilunar valves (*aorta and pulmonary artery*) are similar in
        structure to the cardiac valves.

F. Impulse-conducting system

    1. Modified cardiac muscle fibers specialized for conduction, in
        subendocardial layer.
    2. S. A. node (*pacemaker*), A. V. node, Purkinje fibers (*Bundle of
        His*).

VASCULAR SYSTEM SUMMARIZED

	Tunica Intima (*longitudinal*)	Tunica Media (*circular*)	Tunica Adventitia (*longitudinal*)
Large arteries, > 1 cm	thick, endo-thelium, collagen-ous and elastic fibers	fenestrated elastic membranes, collagen-ous fibers, smooth muscle	thin, collagenous and elastic tissue
Medium arteries, 1 cm-0.5 mm	endothelium, collagenous and elastic fibers, internal elastic membrane	smooth muscle, collagenous and elastic tissue, external elastic membrane	thicker than media, collagenous and elastic tissue
Small arteries, 0.5 mm-20 μ (Arterioles)	endothelium, base-ment membrane, internal elastic membrane	smooth muscle, collagenous and few elastic fibers	loose collagenous tissue
Capillaries, 4-12 μ	endothelium, flat basement membrane, supporting FECT		
Small veins, 20 μ-1 mm (Venules)	endothelium, collagenous fibers	over 45 μ, smooth muscle cells which become continuous layer at 200 μ, FECT	at 300 μ elastic and collagenous tissue
Medium veins, 1 mm-1 cm	endothelium, collagenous and elastic fibers	thin, some smooth muscle, collagenous fibers	thicker than media, smooth muscle, col-lagenous and elastic tissue
Large veins, > 1 cm	endothelium, collagenous and elastic fibers	poorly developed	much thicker than media, elastic and collagenous tissue, smooth muscle

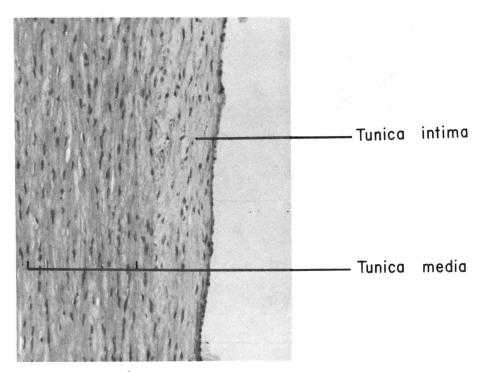

——— Tunica intima

——— Tunica media

Aorta

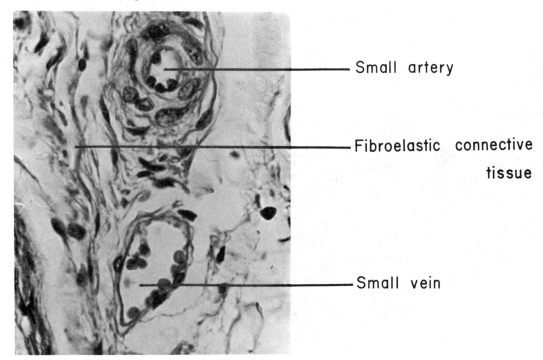

——— Small artery

——— Fibroelastic connective
tissue

——— Small vein

Small Size Artery and Vein

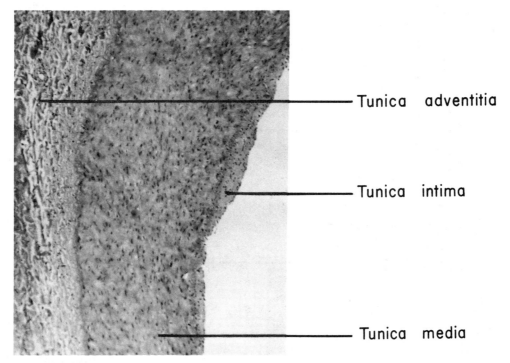

——— Tunica adventitia

——— Tunica intima

——— Tunica media

Medium Size Artery

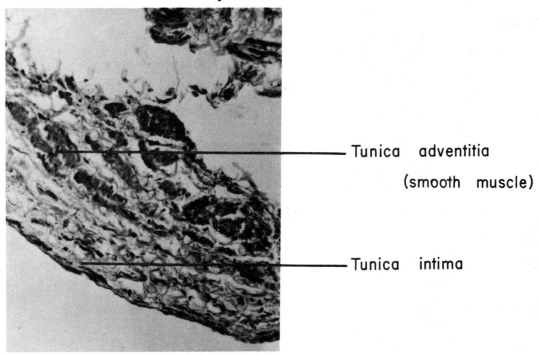

——— Tunica adventitia
(smooth muscle)

——— Tunica intima

Inferior Vena Cava

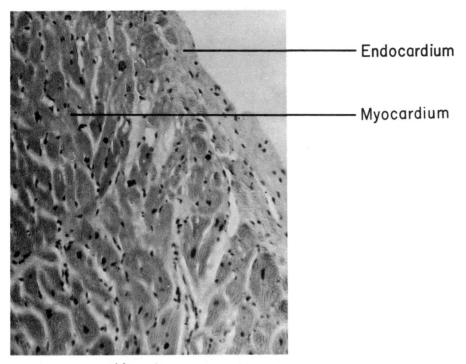

Endocardium

Myocardium

Heart

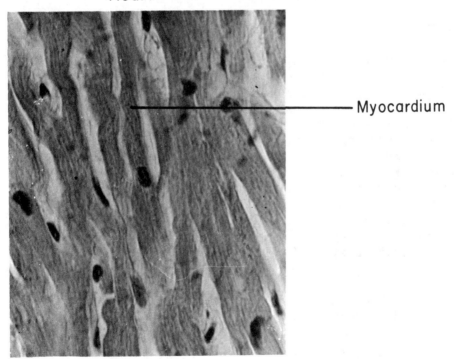

Myocardium

Heart

XI.   LYMPHOID ORGANS

I.   LYMPH DRAINAGE

A.   Vessels

1.   Capillaries - lymphatic
2.   Ducts - lymphatic (*empty to*)
3.   Thoracic duct; empties at junction
     a.   Left subclavian vein, and
     b.   Left internal jugular vein
4.   Right lymphatic duct (*junction*)
     a.   Right subclavian vein
     b.   Right internal jugular vein

II.   LYMPHOID TISSUE

A.   Parenchyma: primarily lymphocytes with some modifications

B.   Stroma: primarily reticular fibers and cells; undifferentiated cells, fixed and free macrophages

III.   LYMPH NODULES

A.   Structural unit (*lymphoid organs*)

1.   Not encapsulated
2.   Cortex - dense small lymphocytes
3.   Antigen → germinal center → proliferating lymphocytes: → small lymphocytes → large lymphocytes → plasma cells → antibody
4.   Transient
5.   Reticulum - dense in cortex
6.   Arteriole and venule supply cortex
7.   Another arteriole and venule supply center
8.   Lymph capillaries not present
9.   Germinal center
     a.   Mitotic cells
     b.   Tingible - body macrophages
     c.   Antigen - trapping dendritic reticular cells
     d.   Large lymphocytes (*immunoblasts*)

IV.   LYMPH NODES

A.   Occurrence and features

1.   Axilla, inguinal, along great vessels of thorax, abdomen, neck, etc.
2.   Bean-shaped body (*1-25 mm*).
3.   Hilus - blood vessels and nerves enter and exit here
4.   Capsule - dense collagenous fibers, scattered elastic fibers, scanty smooth muscle

5. Trabeculae - projections of capsule inwardly
6. Cortex - primarily lymph nodules in circumferential arrangement, sinuses
7. Medulla - irregular arrangement of loose medullary sinuses and denser medullary cords
8. Afferent lymph vessels enter convex surface opposite hilus into the
9. Lymph sinuses (*lined with RE cells*) which drain to
10. Efferent lymph vessels at hilus
11. Reticulum; fibers blend with collagenous fibers of capsule and trabeculae

V. SPLEEN

A. Characteristics

1. Specialized to filter blood
2. No lymph sinuses
3. No afferent lymph vessels
4. Covered by peritoneum except at
5. Hilus; blood vessels enter and exit
6. Capsule - thin, dense, fibrous CT with elastic fibers and some smooth muscle
7. Trabeculae extend inwardly from capsule
8. Parenchyma;
   a. White pulp - lymph nodules with centra artery.
   b. Red pulp
      (1) sinusoids
      (2) cords of Bilroth
9. Reticular fibers (*associated with fixed macrophages*) support the splenic pulp.
10. Vessel arrangement
    a. Arteries
       (1) splenic artery (*enters hilus*).
       (2) trabecular arteries branch off forming
       (3) central arteries, adventitia loosens and becomes a mesh-like reticulum infiltrated with lymphocytes; enlarged areas are splenic nodules.
       (4) after forming capillaries supplying white pulp, the central arteries lose their white pulp investment and enter red pulp to branch and form the
       (5) penicillus - composed of
          (a) pulp arteriole
          (b) sheathed arteriole
          (c) terminal capillary; drains into intercellular spaces or (?) venous sinuses lined with RE cells.
    b. Veins
       (1) venous sinuses lined with phagocytic, reticulo-endothelial cells drain to

(2) pulp veins (*collecting venules*) which unite with
(3) trabecular veins forming the
(4) splenic vein (*hilus exit*).

VI. TONSILS

    A. Palatine

        1. Lymphatic tissue embedded in lamina propria of the mucosa of the oropharynx.
        2. Stratified squamous epithelium (*continuous with mouth and pharynx*).
        3. Capsule - dense fibrous CT at base of organ only.
        4. Trabeculae - form septa.
        5. Reticulum - primarily reticular fibers are continuous with capsule and traberculae.
        6. Crypts - invagination of surface epithelium, well developed.
        7. Lymph nodules - under epithelium and line crypts.
        8. Salivary corpuscles - lymphocytes that migrate through crypt epithelium to saliva.
        9. Mucous glands - outside capsule.
     10. Skeletal muscle is deep and lateral to tonsils.

    B. Lingual

        1. Located on the base of the tongue behind circumvallate papillae.
        2. Stratified squamous epithelium also lines crypts, which are less well developed than in palatine.
        3. Capsule - fibrous CT, not well developed.
        4. Lymph nodules lie between crypts.
        5. Mucous glands frequently open into crypts.

    C. Pharyngeal

        1. "Adenoids" - located in nasopharynx
        2. Pseudostratified ciliated columnar epithelium
        3. Capsule - fibrous CT, not well developed
        4. Lymphatic tissue is similar to palatine type.
        5. Lymph nodules in folds - not crypts.
        6. Mixed sero-mucous glands

VII. THYMUS

    A. Characteristics

        1. Two lobes united by CT
        2. Capsule - surrounding each lobe
        3. Septa - invagination of capsule
        4. Lobules - formed by septa
        5. Each lobule - cortex and medulla

6. Cortex - reticular meshwork with lymphocytes (*thymocytes*)
7. No lymph nodules
8. Thymic (*Hassall's*) corpuscles form from reticular cells formed from entoderm. Appearance is similar to a cross-section of onion.
9. No afferent lymph vessels
10. No lymph sinuses

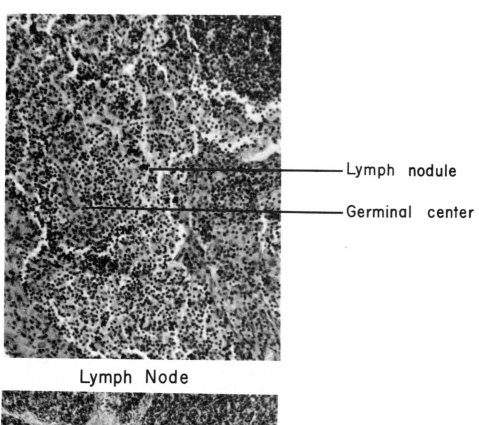

Lymph nodule

Germinal center

Lymph Node

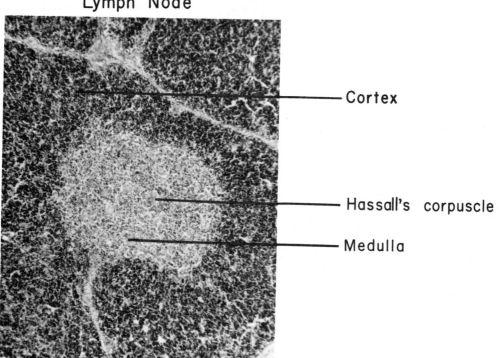

Cortex

Hassall's corpuscle

Medulla

Thymus

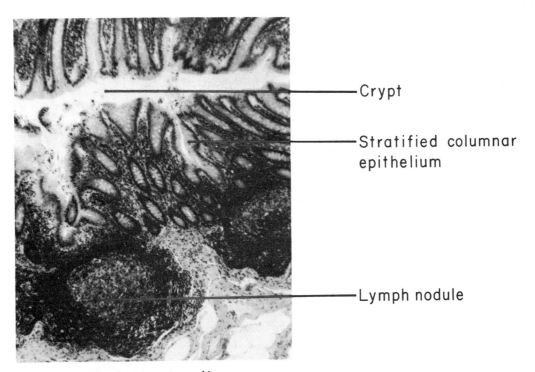

Crypt

Stratified columnar epithelium

Lymph nodule

Palatine tonsil

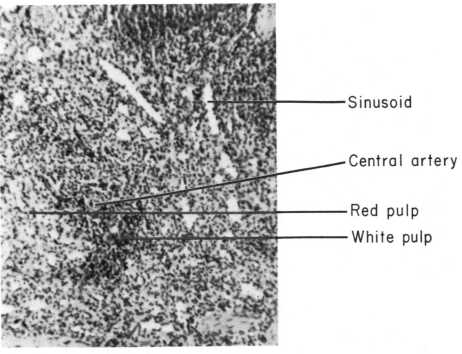

Sinusoid

Central artery

Red pulp

White pulp

Spleen

XII. THE INTEGUMENT

I. SKIN

   A. Epidermis

      1. Stratified squamous epithelium derived from ectoderm
      2. Cell layers (*palms and soles*)
         a. Stratum malpighii
            (1) stratum germinativum (*basal cell layer*) - an active
               and proliferative single layer of basophilic columnar
               or cuboidal cells anchored in the underlying dermal
               CT by short cytoplasmic processes.
            (2) stratum spinosum - proliferative cells are several
               layers thick, basophilic and have cytoplasmic projec-
               tions forming desmosomes. Tonofibrils (*with tono-
               filaments*) attach to the cell membrane at desmosome
               sites. Tonofilaments may represent the first stage
               in the production of the fibrous protein keratin in
               keratinocytes.
         b. Stratum granulosum - flattened cells, 3 to 5 layers thick,
           with dark nuclei. Keratohyaline granules are found
           about the tonofilaments in the cytoplasm. Cells die in
           this stratum.
         c. Stratum lucidum - a translucent layer, 3 to 5 cell layers
           thick, cell entities indistinct. Cytoplasm contains a
           semifluid substance called eleidin which may represent
           a form of keratin.
         d. Stratum corneum - the anucleate cells form broad flat
           scales whose edges interdigitate with each other. Cyto-
           plasm is replaced by soft keratin (*low in sulphur content
           as opposed to hard keratin of nails and hair cortex*). The
           scales desquamate constantly.
      3. Melanocytes
         a. Melanocytes differentiate from melanoblasts of the neural
           crest; they appear as clear cells in an H & E section
           scattered in the basal layer in a ratio approaching 1:12.
           Positive identification of melanocytes is made with
           dihydroxyphenylalanine (DOPA) which blackens these cells.
         b. Melanin is formed in a melanosome (*intracellular particle
           0.3 to 0.7 μ D*); it is deposited on concentric dense sheets
           which are covered by a membrane.
      4. Langerhans cells of the stratum spinosum may be macrophages.

   B. Dermis

      1. Dense irregularly arranged CT (*0.5 mm to 3 mm D*) extending
        from the basal cell layer to the hypodermis. Two strata are
        present:
         a. Papillary layer
            (1) composed of fine FECT whose reticular fibers form a
               basement membrane beneath the basal cell layer; the

processes of the basal cells anchor in the fibers of
the membrane. Some papillae contain special nerve
terminations; others, capillary loops.
    b. Reticular layer
      (1) composed of coarse FECT whose fibers course parallel
to the surface forming lines of skin tension termed
Langer's lines; these are important surgically.
  2. Cellular elements
    a. Fibroblasts and macrophages predominate.
    b. Smooth muscle cell bundles (*arrector pili*)
    c. Some striated muscle cells

C. Hypodermis (*superficial fascia*)

  1. Is fatty, areolar CT beneath, and inseparable from, the dermis.
When the fat cells are abundant, the fat layer is known
as the panniculus adiposus.

II. HAIR

A. Shaft and root

  1. Hairs grow out of epithelial pockets - hair follicles.
  2. Hairs are composed of epithelial cells arranged in three concentric layers:
    a. Medulla
      (1) axis of 2 or 3 layers of cuboidal cells containing
keratohyaline granules and shrunken nuclei.
    b. Cortex
      (1) forms the greater portion of the hair with several
layers of flattened cells with hard keratin. Melanocytes present are responsible for hair color. Accu-
mulation of intercellular air spaces results in gray-
ing hair along with absence of pigment.
    c. Cuticle
      (1) is formed by a single layer of transparent enucleated
cells forming keratinized scales.
  3. Appearance
    a. Straight hair - round
    b. Wavy hair - oval
    c. Wooly - elliptical
  4. Root
    a. Lies in hair follicle.
    b. Hair bulb is the lower knoblike expansion of the root.

B. Hair follicle

  1. (*Inner*) epithelial root sheath (*derived from epidermis*) surrounds the hair shaft below the sebaceous gland and is composed of three layers:

      a. Cuticle of root sheath
         (1) interlocks with and lies against the hair cuticle;
              similar to it in structure.
      b. Huxley's layer
         (1) contains several rows of elongated cells with tri-
              chohyaline (*eleidin-like granules*).
      c. Henle's layer
         (1) is a single row of flattened clear cells containing
              hyaline fibrils.

  2. Outer epithelial root sheath is a continuation of the stratum
      germinativum.

  3. CT sheath consists of three layers:
      a. Inner (*glassy membrane*)
         (1) of reticular fibers and amorphous ground substance;
              corresponds to the basement membrane beneath the
              epidermis.
      b. Middle
         (1) is thick and contains circularly arranged fine CT
              fibers; corresponds to the papillary layer of the
              dermis.
      c. Outer
         (1) poorly defined and consists of coarse collagen fibers
              (*longitudinal*); corresponds to the reticular layer of
              the dermis.

III. NAILS

  A. Structure

    1. Nail plate
      a. Body
         (1) flattened cornified epithelial cells with shrunken
              nuclei; analogous to the stratum corneum.
      b. Free edge
         (1) epidermis below is the hyponychium.
      c. Root
         (1) nail matrix
            (a) lies beneath the root; it is a thickened stratum
                germinativum whose cells proliferate and dif-
                ferentiate to provide the forward growth of the
                nail.
      d. Lunula
         (1) crescentric opaque proximal junction of body and
              root.

    2. Nail fold
      a. Has the structure of skin.
      b. Cuticle or eponychium is the ordinary stratum corneum
        growing over the lunula.

    3. Nail groove
      a. Is the cleft between the body and the fold.

4. Nail bed
    a. Is the deeper layers of the epidermis covered by the body, and covering a highly vascular dermis.

IV. GLANDS

A. Sebaceous glands

1. Are connected to hair follicles except at lip margin, in the nipple, glans and prepuce of the penis and the labia majora. They are lacking in the palms and soles.
2. Are simple or branched alveolar glands of holocrine type, and are encapsulated in CT in the dermis.
3. The excretory duct empties into the neck of the follicle; it is lined with stratified cuboidal (or *squamous*) epithelium continuous with the outer root sheath and stratum germinativium as well as the peripheral cells of the alveolus.
4. The peripheral cells are low cuboidal, small, and mitotically active. They become progressively larger toward the interior as fat droplets accumulate in them.
5. The interior cells apparently disintegrate, produce sebum, and are replaced by peripheral cells. Sebum discharge seems to be aided by the arrector pili muscle.

B. Sweat glands

1. Eccrine sweat glands are distributed throughout the skin except in the lip margin, nail bed, glans penis, and ear drum.
2. They are simple, coiled, tubular glands with the secretory part deep in the dermis or hypodermis.
3. The excretory duct opens on the surface by the sweat pore. The coiled secretory duct is lined by simple columnar or cuboidal epithelium on a distinct basement membrane; nuclei are round, cytoplasmic vacuolated, and contain fat droplets.
4. Myoepithelial cells are between the bases of cells and the basement membrane; they spiral longitudinally around the tubule, and may aid in emptying the glandular secretion.
5. The secretory duct narrows into a thin excretory duct. The wall of the duct consists of stratified cuboidal epithelium on a delicate basement membrane which is surrounded by FECT. No myoepithelial cells are present.
6. Apocrine sweat glands are especially large and found in the axilla, mammary areola, labia majora, on the scrotum, and the public and circumanal regions. They are branched, tubular glands. Apocrine sweat glands also include the ceruminous glands of the external auditory canals, and the glands of Moll in the eyelid margin.
7. Mammary glands are described in the "Female Reproduction System".

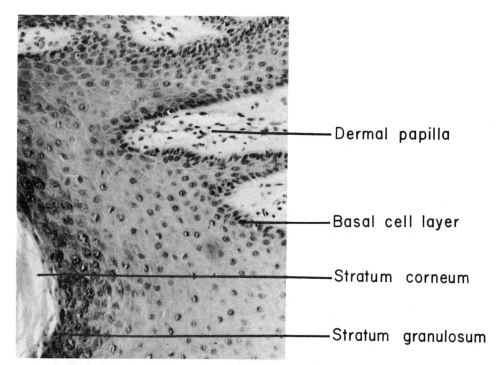

— Dermal papilla

— Basal cell layer

— Stratum corneum

— Stratum granulosum

Thick Skin

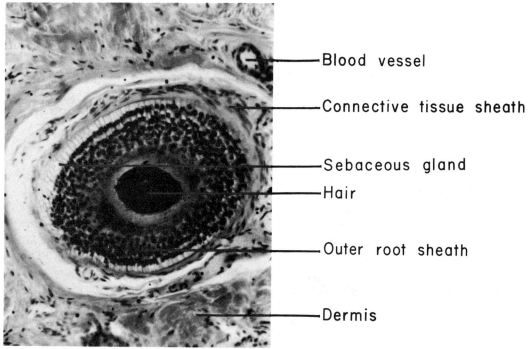

— Blood vessel

— Connective tissue sheath

— Sebaceous gland

— Hair

— Outer root sheath

— Dermis

Cross-section of a Hair Follicle

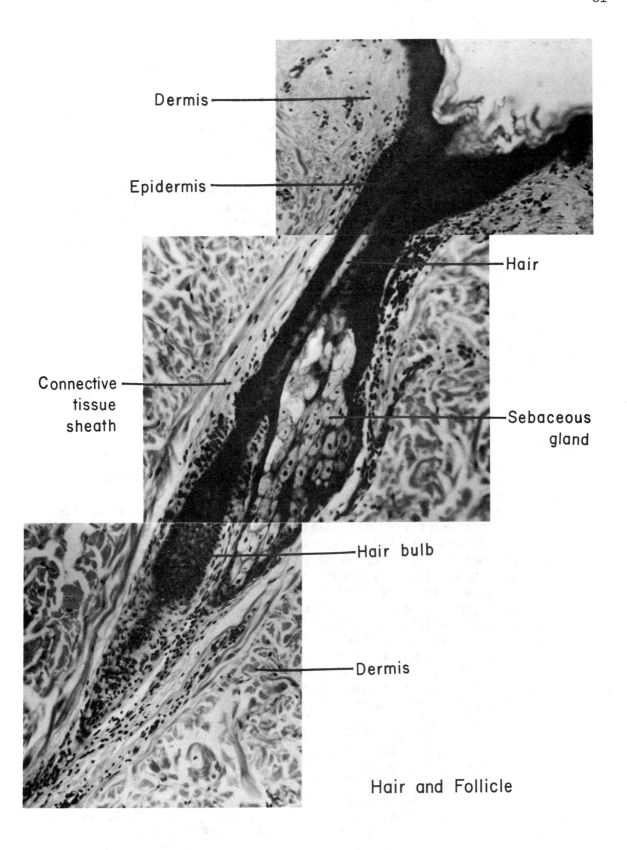

Dermis

Epidermis

Hair

Connective
tissue
sheath

Sebaceous
gland

Hair bulb

Dermis

Hair and Follicle

XIII. THE DIGESTIVE SYSTEM

I. THE ORAL CAVITY

   A. The lip

      1. The oral cavity is lined with a mucous membrane lying on a
         vascular FECT layer. The mucosa consists of
         a. Stratified squamous epithelium.
         b. Basement membrane.
         c. Lamina propria.
      2. The lip is composed of a core of skeletal muscle (*obicularis
         oris*) cells embedded in FECT, and covered externally by skin;
         an internal poorly keratinized, modified, stratified squamous
         epithelium lies on a lamina propria with high papillae; within
         the lamina propria are mixed and mucous glands. The dermis
         has a rich plexus of capillaries which are prominent at the
         free margin of the lip.

   B. The cheek

      1. The cheek has a structure similar to the lip. One exception
         is the abundant elastic fibers present in the submucosa.
         These are continuous with the fibers surrounding the striated
         muscle and the lamina propria. This arrangement gives a
         maximum of distensibility to the oral mucous membrane.

   C. The tongue

      1. The tongue is composed primarily of a core of skeletal muscle
         and glands, and is covered by a mucous membrane.
      2. The anterior 2/3 of the upper oral portion is separated from
         the posterior 1/3 pharyngeal portion by the
         a. Sulcus terminalis.
      3. Lingual papillae appear on the oral portion as surface pro-
         jections. They are formed of a central core of CT lamina
         propria covered by stratified squamous epithelium. Three
         types present according to shape:
         a. Circumvallate papillae
            (1) are located along the sulcus terminalis as projections
                surrounded by a moat. Taste buds are present on the
                lateral walls. Ducts of von Ebner's glands (*serous*)
                open into the circular furrow (*moat*).
         b. Filiform papillae
            (1) most numerous of all the papillae with a conical ap-
                pearance; quite evenly distributed over the entire
                oral upper portion.
         c. Fungiform papillae
            (1) relatively few in number, and are interspersed singly
                among the parallel rows of the filiform papillae;
                they have a mushroom appearance. Taste buds are pre-
                sent only on the oral surface of the epithelium in

contradistinction to the position of taste buds on
the circumvallate papillae whose taste buds are primarily in the lateral walls.
   d. Folliate papillae
     (1) rudimentary in humans, but well developed in lower
        animals.
4. The pharyngeal portion is free of papillae, but contains the
   the lingual tonsils.
5. Other than von Ebner's glands, mixed glands of Nühn are
   located in the anterior portion. Their ducts open into the
   crypts of the lingual tonsils, and dorsal surface of the
   tongue.
6. Taste buds
   a. Appear as pale, barrel-like bodies in papillae, and a few
     are also present on the palate and epiglottis. The two
     kinds of cells present are
     (1) supporting cells which are spindle-shaped, and are
        arranged like barrel staves to surround the inner
        taste pore at the base.
     (2) neuroepithelial taste cells are distributed between
        the supporting cells. Each cell is long and slender
        with an elongated central nucleus, and terminates as
        short taste hair which projects into the external
        opening, the
        (a) outer taste pore.

D. The teeth

1. Development
   a. Dental primordium
     (1) formed from basal cells of the oral ectoderm.
   b. Labiodental lamina
     (1) an epithelial shelf that grows from the thickened
        primordium into the mesenchyme as a bifid structure.
        The external limb splits later to form a groove that
        deepens to separate the lip and the remainder of the
        mouth. The internal limb is the dental lamina.
        Cells proliferate to form five tooth-buds (*germs*) in
        each half-jaw. Later a second set of tooth-buds de-
        velops on the lingual side of each developing de-
        ciduous tooth plus three more posteriorly in each
        half-jaw. With further differentiation, the bell-
        shaped epithelial bud becomes the
   c. Enamel organ
     (1) which forms enamel, and caps the
   d. Dental papilla
     (1) the condensation of mesenchyme which gives rise to
        dentin and pulp.
   e. Dental sac (*follicle*)
     (1) a CT sac surrounds the enamel organ and dental papilla
        that forms cementum and the peridontal membrane.

       f.   Stellate reticulum
          (1)   central cells of enamel organ.
       g.   Ameloblasts
          (1)   tall columnar cells of the inner enamel epithelium adjacent to the dental papilla which form enamel.
       h.   Odontoblasts (*dentinoblasts*)
          (1)   peripheral tall columnar cells of the dental papilla which form dentin.
2.   Structure
       a.   Crown - above gum margin.
       b.   Root - 1 to 3 cm below gum margin.
       c.   Alveolus - root socket in jaw bone.
       d.   Neck - root and crown meet.
       e.   Periodontal membrane - attaches root to alveolar wall.
       f.   Pulp chamber - extends from crown into root canals.
       g.   Apical foramen - canal opening at tip of root.
       h.   Dental pulp - soft core of loosely arranged CT occupying the chamber.
       i.   Tooth wall
          (1)   dentin - borders pulp.
          (2)   enamel - covers crown, and thins at neck.
          (3)   cementum - encrusts root, and thins at neck.
3.   Dentin
       a.   Odontoblasts form the dentin matrix throughout the life of a tooth.
          (1)   amorphous intercellular substance
             (a)   72% inorganic salts
             (b)   28% organic material
          (2)   Korff's fibers
             (a)   reticular fibers formed in predentin (*uncalcified dentin*).
          (3)   as intercellular substance continues to form, collagenic fibers replace reticular fibers.
       b.   Tomes' dentinal fibers (*odontoblastic processes*)
          (1)   cytoplasmic extensions of the odontoblasts continuing through the predentin and dentinal layers to the dentin-enamel junction. They occupy a space in the dentin matrix known as
       c.   Dentinal tubules
          (1)   which course from pulp cavity to dentin periphery in an S form giving dentin a radially striated appearance.
       d.   Increment lines (*of Ebner and Owen*)
          (1)   represent layered deposits of dentin resembling growth rings in a tree.
4.   Enamel
       a.   Ameloblasts form enamel which covers only the tooth crown.
          (1)   96% inorganic salts
             (a)   about 90% is calcium phosphate in the form of apatite crystals.

        (2) 4% organic material and water
     b. Enamel prism
        (1) each prism is formed by one ameloblast.
     c. Increment lines (of Retzius).
        (1) periods of rhythmic growth
  5. Pulp
     a. Originates from the dental papilla containing condensed mesenchyme.
     b. Consists of fibroblasts, macrophages, peripheral odontoblasts, reticular fibers, and nerve fibers, and blood vessels which pass via the apical foramen.
  6. Cementum
     a. Cells of the dental sac differentiate into cementoblasts which deposit cementum on the dentin of the root from neck to apex. Cementum has coarse collagen fibers (Sharpey's) in a bone-like calcified matrix.
  7. Periodontal membrane
     a. CT formed from dental sac with fibroblasts, osteoblasts, cementoblasts, collagen fibers, blood vessels, and nerve fibers
     b. It attaches the root to
        (1) alveolar wall
        (2) gingival CT
        (3) roots (superficial parts) of other teeth
     c. Sharpey's fibers
        (1) extend from cementum to alveolar wall via the membrane.
  8. Gingiva (gum)
     a. Resembles somewhat the epidermis of the skin.
     b. Gingival crest (unattached)
     c. Gingival sulcus
        (1) epithelial attachment
           (a) at the bottom of the sulcus the gingival epithelium adheres to the tooth. The epithelium extends below the enamel to the cementum which is covered by a PAS positive membrane which provides the same means of attachment for materials as basement membranes elsewhere.

II. SALIVARY GLANDS

A. Major

  1. Parotid
     a. A compound tubulo-alveolar, serous gland of the merocrine type situated below and anterior to the ear.
     b. A well-developed CT capsule gives off septa dividing the gland into lobes and lobules. Septal CT often contains fat cells. The CT surrounding acini and ducts contains capillaries, and nerve fibers.

    c. Acinar cells are large and pyramidal with basal nuclei;
       acini are elongated and enclosed in a basement membrane
       with myoepithelial (*basket*) cells.

    d. Intercalated ducts are lined with simple cuboidal cells
       continuous with acini cells.

    e. The striated duct (*intralobular*) is formed of simple
       columnar cells with basal striations. It is the next order
       of ducts following the intercalated duct. The striated
       duct joins

    f. Excretory ducts (*interlobular*) composed at first of simple
       columnar cells which become increasingly tall along the
       course of the excretory duct system until finally becoming
       lined with stratified columnar epithelium in the larger
       ducts. The major duct (*Stenson's*) opens opposite the
       second upper molar.

    g. Sensory innervation by the fifth nerve
       (1) secretory (*motor*)
          (a) sympathetic, superior cervical ganglion (*vaso-
              constriction*)
          (b) parasympathetic, ninth nerve, otic ganglion
              (*vasodilation*)

2. Submandibular

    a. A tubulo-alveolar, merocrine gland (*mixed*) with primarily
       serous acini, demilunes.

    b. It has a CT capsule, septa, and a duct system similar to
       those of the parotid gland.

    c. Acini rest on a basement membrane with some myoepithelial
       cells present.

    d. Intercalated ducts are short and lined with simple cuboidal
       epithelium leading to secretory (*striated*) ducts and ex-
       cretory ducts.

    e. Submandibular (*Wharton's*) duct is lined with stratified
       columnar epithelium, and opens on the frontal-lateral
       margin of the frenulum linguae.

    f. Sensory innervation by the fifth nerve
       (1) secretory (*motor*)
          (a) sympathetic, superior cervical ganglion (*vaso-
              constriction*)
          (b) parasympathetic, seventh nerve, chorda tympani,
              submandibular ganglion (*vasodilation*)

3. Sublingual

    a. A collection of glands located under the mucous membrane
       of the floor of the mouth. The largest is a tubulo-
       alveolar merocrine gland (*mixed*) with mostly mucous acini
       bearing serous demilunes.

    b. No definite capsule, but with septa, and some myoepithelial
       cells.

    c. Intercalated and striated ducts are rare or absent.

    d. The largest, sublingual, is drained by the ductus sub-
       lingualis major (*Bartholin's*) which empties on the side of
       the frenulum linguae; the duct is of stratified columnar
       epithelium.

      e. Innervation is the same as that of the submandibular
         gland.

B. Minor

    1. Palatine
      a. Located between the mucous membrane and the bone in the
         hard palate, and extends posteriorly and laterally
      b. Long, branched tubulo-alveolar mixed glands, primarily
         mucous.
    2. Buccal
      a. Embedded in the mucous membrane of the cheeks; mixed
         glands, but mostly mucous.
    3. Labial
      a. Anterior continuations of the buccal glands.
    4. Lingual
      a. Anterior lingual (*Blandin-Nühn*), embedded within muscula-
         ture of inferior aspect of tongue near the tip. Chiefly
         mucous.
      b. Posterior lingual
         (1) glands of the circumvallate papillae (*von Ebner's*)
         (2) glands of the base of the tongue; pure mucous.

C. Saliva

    1. Among the constituents comprising saliva such things as mucin,
       glycoprotein and salivary enzymes are synthesized by the paren-
       chyma and therefore are an intrinsic function of the glandular
       cells. Other substances including electrolytes, blood group
       proteins, and gamma globulins represent a spill-over from
       blood during the formation of saliva.

D. Palate

    1. Hard palate
      a. Oral mucous membrane is composed of stratified squamous,
         keratinized epithelium underlying lamina propria which
         blends with the periosteum of the bone. Fat cells and
         mixed glands exhibit in the lamina propria which is thin
         in the midline and attached to a median, bony ridge - the
         raphe.
    2. Soft palate
      a. Layers from the oral surface
         (1) stratified squamous, nonkeratinizing epithelium (*or
            pseudostratified ciliated columnar epithelium on
            respiratory surface*)
         (2) lamina propria - has a few glands and forms a strong
            aponeurosis near the hard palate.
         (3) muscle layer - skeletal

* COMPARISON OF THE MAJOR SALIVARY GLANDS

	Parotid	Submandibular	Sublingual
Size and shape	Largest; main and accessory parts both encapsulated; compound, branched, alveolar	Intermediate; well limited and encapsulated; compound, branched, alveolar, partly tubular	Smallest; major gland and several minor ones; no capsule; compound, branched, tubuloalveolar
Position	Filling retromandibular fossa and reaches around mandibular ramus anterior to ear	Beneath mandible	In floor of mouth
Ducts	Parotid (Stensen's) duct opens opposite second upper molar; double layer columnar cells on marked basement membrane	Submandibular (Wharton's) duct opens on either side of frenulum of tongue; structure same	Major sublingual (Bartholin's) duct opens near submandibular sometimes by common aperture, also several minor sublingual (Rivinian) ducts; structure same
Secretory ducts	Single layer very conspicuously striated columnar cells	Same but somewhat longer and may contain yellow pigment	Rare or absent
Intercalated ducts	Long, narrow, branching made of single layer of flattened cells	Much shorter but similar structure	Absent
Secretory epithelium	Serous alveoli, mucous alveoli rare (in newborn infant)	Serous alveoli predominate, some mucous alveoli have serous crescents	Major gland: mucous alveoli predominate; many serous crescents and alveoli Minor glands all mucous
Interstitial tissue	Fat cells most abundant		Connective tissue septa most abundant
Nerve supply	Sensory: fifth nerve Secretory: (1) sympathetic, superior cervical ganglion (vasoconstriction); (2) parasympathetic, ninth nerve, otic ganglion (vasodilation)	Sensory: fifth nerve Secretory: (1) sympathetic, same; (2) parasympathetic, seventh nerve, chorda tympani, submandibular ganglion (vasodilation)	Sensory: fifth nerve Secretory: same as submandibular gland

* From Finerty, J. C. and Cowdry, E. V. A Textbook of Histology. 5th edition, Table 25, p. 369, Lea & Febiger, Philadelphia. 1960.

III. TUBULAR DIGESTIVE TRACT

   A. General plan

       1. Mucosa membrane (*tunica mucosa*)
         a. Moist surface epithelium
         b. Basement membrane
         c. Lamina propria delicate
            (1) loose, areolar CT
         d. Muscularis mucosae
            (1) when present it may have an inner circular layer and
            (2) outer longitudinal layer.
         e. Villi (*evaginations of mucosa*)
         f. Mucosal glands or crypts (*invaginations of mucosa*)
       2. Submucosa (*tunica submucosa*)
         a. Coarse areolar CT
            (1) plexuses of nerves and ganglion cells termed
                Meissner's plexus
            (2) some areas may contain glands (*Brunner's glands*) in
                duodenum.
       3. Muscularis externa (*tunica muscularis*)
         a. Inner circular layer
          b. Outer longitudinal smooth muscle layer
          c. Auerbach's myenteric plexus
            (1) between the inner and outer muscle layers is a plexus
                of nerves associated with numerous ganglion cells.
       4. Adventitia
         a. Outermost, dense areolar CT containing blood vessels,
           nerves, and lymphatics
         b. Serosa
            (1) adventitia plus peritoneum (*mesothelium*)

   B. The esophagus

       1. Mucous membrane
         a. Moist stratified squamous (*nonkeratinized*) epithelium
         b. Lamina propria
            (1) loose areolar CT with some lymphatic nodules,
                and scattered lymphocytes
            (2) cardiac glands - mucous glands in upper and lower
                1/3 of esophagus
         c. Muscularis mucosae
            (1) thick; replaces the elastic layer of the pharynx
                at the cricoid cartilage level. Incomplete
                bundles in upper 1/3; complete in middle and
                lower 1/3.
       2. Submucosa
         a. Thick, with coarse collagenous fibers and mucous glands
           termed esophageal glands.

3. Muscularis externa
   a. Arises at the level of the cricoid cartilage. In the
      upper third there are skeletal muscle cells only, both
      skeletal and smooth in the middle third, and the lower
      third has only smooth muscle cells.
4. Adventitia
   a. Is loose CT with blood vessels, nerves, and lymphatics.
5. Diagram:

	epithelium	muscularis mucosa	glands	muscularis externa
upper 1/3	moist strati- fied squamous	incomplete	cardiac & esophageal	skeletal
middle 1/3	moist strati- fied squamous	complete	esophageal	smooth & skeletal
lower 1/3	moist strati- fied squamous	complete	cardiac & esophageal	smooth

C. The stomach

1. Mucous membrane
   a. Simple columnar epithelium with apical mucous
   b. Lamina propria
      (1) highly vascular, cellular, sometimes lymph nodules
          present, and contains gastric glands.
   c. Muscularis mucosae
      (1) smooth muscle fibers extend up around glands.
2. Submucosa
   a. Coarse collagenous bundles, elastic fibers, blood vessels,
      lymph vessels, Meissner's plexus, and fat cells.
3. Muscularis externa
   a. Inner oblique layer
   b. Middle circular layer
   c. Outer longitudinal layer
4. Serosa
5. Gastric glands
   a. Cardiac glands
      (1) ring-shaped area in the immediate vicinity of the
          cardia.
      (2) simple or branched tubular, several may open into
          each foveola or gastric pit base.
      (3) the pale columnar cells secrete mucous (*similar to
          mucous neck cells of fundic stomach*), and are inter-
          spersed with a few parietal cells.

    b. Fundic glands
       (1) pits extend to 1/3 of the mucosal thickness, and the glands are long and branched.
       (2) four cell types are present:
           (a) surface mucous cells are high columnar and cover the entire surface and line the foveolae. Cuboidal shaped at the neck of gland.
           (b) mucous neck cells are located in the upper ends of the gland interspersed among parietal cells, and are smaller than surface cells. Increase mitosis in this area.
           (c) parietal or oxyntic cells are large and acidophilic. Secretory canaliculi may be visible at the apex where HCl is secreted, pyramidal shaped.
           (d) chief (*zymogenic*) cells are located in the lower portions of the gland, basophilic, and contains pepsinogen, precursor of pepsin. Zymogen granules in apical end. Rennin and gastric intrinsic (*anti-pernicious anemia*) factor may be produced by chief cells. A few argentaffin cells may be demonstrated among chief cells: They may secrete serotonin, a vasoconstrictor substance.
    c. Pyloric glands
       (1) pits extend 3/4 to muscularis mucosa; lined by mucous, columnar epithelium
       (2) glands lined by cells similar to mucous neck cells with a few parietal cells interspersed.
       (3) coiled

D. The small intestine
   1. Duodenum
   2. Jejunum
   3. Ileum
   4. Mucosal surface modifications:
     a. Plicae circulares (*valves of Kerkring*) are spiral folds of the mucosa and submucosa.
     b. Villi and crypts
       (1) villi (*projections of mucosa*) are covered by epithelium and have a core of lamina propria. They are broad in the duodenum, but finger-like in the ileum. Strands of smooth muscle extend into the villus from the muscularis mucosae.
       (2) crypts (*glands of Lieberkühn*) are tubelike structures opening between the bases of villi and nearly reach the muscularis mucosae, as invaginations of mucosa. The base of a crypt is lined with a cluster of Paneth cells.
     c. Microvilli are present on columnar absorptive cells covering villi and lining crypts, a striated border.

5. Epithelium
   a. Types
      (1) simple columnar absorptive cells with striated border (*microvilli*).
      (2) undifferentiated columnar cells in the crypt, with increased mitosis.
      (3) goblet cells produce mucus and are scattered between columnar cells. Increase from duodenum to ileum.
      (4) argentaffin cells are scattered singly in the crypts, (*which apparently produce serotonin*).
      (5) paneth cells with acidophilic granules lie in clusters at the bottom of crypts, apparently produce enzymes.
6. Lamina propria
   a. Extends between the crypts and into the core of the villi. Cellular elements include primitive reticular cells with large oval, pale nuclei; lymphocytes, eosinophils, plasma cells, macrophages, and smooth muscle cells. Also capillaries and lacteals. In the ileum aggregated nodules of lymphoid tissue exhibit as Peyer's patches, but solitary lymphoid follicles appear in other areas of small intestine.
7. Muscularis mucosae
8. Submucosa
   a. Brunner's glands appear in the first 1/4 of the duodenum and are mucus secreting. They open into the crypts of Lieberkühn.
   b. In the region of Peyer's patches this layer is usually infiltrated with lymphocytes.
9. Muscularis externa
10. Serosa

E. Appendix (*mucosa is similar to large intestine, muscularis externa like small intestine*).
   1. Villi are absent, crypts are present with few Paneth cells but numerous argentaffin cells.
   2. Mucosa surface epithelium is of columnar cells with striated borders. Lamina propria contains lymphoid tissue, and the muscularis mucosa usually is incomplete, due to heavy lymphocytic infiltration.
   3. Submucosa is thick and contains blood vessels and nerves.
   4. Muscularis externa exhibits two layers.
   5. Serosa.

F. The large intestine

   1. Lacks plicae and villi, but crypts are present.
   2. Epithelial cell types are similar, but goblet cells are more numerous than in the small intestine.
   3. Ileocecal junction.

     4. Cecum, colon, and rectum
        a. Crypts are long and closely packed, goblet cells are numerous, argentaffin and Paneth cells are scarce. Lamina propria appears similar to that in the small intestine, and the muscularis mucosae is well-developed.
        b. The outer layer of the muscularis externa appears incomplete as three bands, taeniae coli; in the rectum it again becomes complete.

  G. Rectoanal junction
     1. Only crypts.
     2. Transitional area of simple columnar in rectum, to moist stratified squamous to dry stratified squamous at external orifice.
     3. Muscularis mucosa fans out into adjacent FECT at rectoanal junction.
     4. Muscularis externa "proliferates" into internal anal sphincter.

IV. MAJOR DIGESTIVE GLANDS

  A. Pancreas

     1. Is a lobulated, compound, tubulo-alveolar gland, has both an exocrine and endocrine secretory function
     2. No organized capsule, but has a thin layer of loose CT from which septa pass internally dividing the gland into many small lobules. The delicate CT contains blood vessels, lymphatics, nerves, and excretory ducts.
     3. Duct of Wirsung is the main excretory duct, and duct of Santorini is the smaller accessory duct.
     4. The larger and interlobular ducts are lined with simple columnar epithelium and with goblet cells.
     5. Intercalated ducts arising within the lobules from the continued branching of the interlobulated ducts are lined by low cuboidal cells.
     6. Centroacinar cells form a truncated cuboidal epithelium within the lumen of acini and are continuous with the epithelium of the intercalated duct.
     7. Acini are serous. Acinar cells have a basal zone which is basophilic and an apical zone with zymogen granules which are probably the precursors of the enzymes in pancreatic secretion; trypsin, chymotrypsin, amylase, and lipase.
     8. Islet of Langerhans
        a. Endocrine cell aggregations which are interspersed irregularly among the acini.
        b. Cells
           (1) A or alpha cells have fine cytoplasmic granules, and are presumed to form glucagon.
           (2) B or beta cells have coarse cytoplasmic granules, are more numerous than A cells, and produce insulin.

(3) D or delta cells whose significance is uncertain.

B. The liver

1. Glisson's thin capsule of FECT covers the surface except at
    the diaphragmatic attachment, CT septa extend from the cap-
    sule forming lobes, and lobules, hepatic lobule
    a. Epithelial parenchyma is composed of hepatic cells irregu-
        larly arranged in plates seen on edge as cell cords. The
        cords are radially arranged about the central vein.
    b. Afferent blood vessels are the portal vein and hepatic
        artery both of which give off interlobular branches
        (1) branches from the portal vein enter the lobule and
             empty into the hepatic sinusoids; they converge toward
             the center to empty into the central vein, an effer-
             ent vessel. Central veins unite to form a sublobular
             vein, a branch of the hepatic vein.
        (2) the hepatic artery follows the branching of the por-
             tal vein through the interlobular CT. Interlobular
             arterioles empty into the hepatic sinusoids, which
             drain to the central vein.
    c. Hepatic cells are polyhedral in form with a central
        nucleus, one or more nucleoli; and cytoplasm which may
        contain glycogen, fat droplets, and pigment granules.
        Stellate cells of von Kupffer are macrophages seen lining
        hepatic sinusoids. The space of Disse separates hepatic
        cells from endothelial cells, and is active in transfer
        between blood and parenchyma.
2. Bile is produced by hepatic cells (*exocrine function*), and
    bile ducts transport it to the duodenum. Bile canaliculi are
    located between hepatic cells and are usually too small to
    see with the light microscope. The canaliculi empty into
    interlobular ducts, part of the triad.
3. Functions of liver include:
    a. Removal of bile pigments from blood which are excreted in
        bile.
    b. Storing of glycogen.
    c. Converting fats, and perhaps proteins, to carbohydrates
        (*gluconeogenesis*).
    d. Maintaining constancy of blood glucose level.
    e. Being chief site of amino acid deamination with urea as a
        by-product.
    f. Metabolizing fat and storing in the liver.
    g. Synthesizing plasma proteins such as fibrinogen, pro-
        thrombin, and albumin.
    h. Storing of essential vitamins (A, D, B_2, B_3, B_4, B_{12}, and
        K).
    i. Being an embryonic hemopoietic organ.

C. The gallbladder

    1. Structure
        a. Fundus
        b. Body
        c. Neck
            (1) mucosal folds form the spiral valve of Heister.
        d. Wall
            (1) mucosa
                (a) epithelium is tall columnar with a striated border.
                (b) lamina propria of CT has extensive vascular plexuses and may contain a few smooth muscle cells.
                (c) Rokitansky-Aschoff sinuses are small diverticula of the mucosa which extend into the muscular and perimuscular layers, and may indicate pathological change.
            (2) muscularis externa
                (a) layers of smooth muscle separated by layers of CT.
            (3) serosa
                (a) a broad perimuscular CT coat, rich in blood and lymphatic vessels, and elastic fibers.
    2. Bile ducts
        a. Cystic duct
        b. Hepatic duct
        c. Common bile duct
        d. Mucosa
            (1) ducts are lined by columnar epithelium, with goblet cells.
        e. Muscularis externa
            (1) no definite pattern.

96

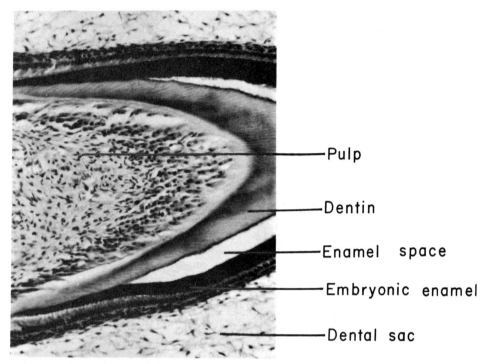

Pulp

Dentin

Enamel space

Embryonic enamel

Dental sac

Developing Tooth

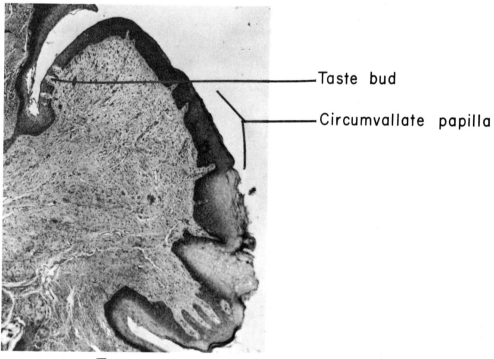

Taste bud

Circumvallate papilla

Tongue

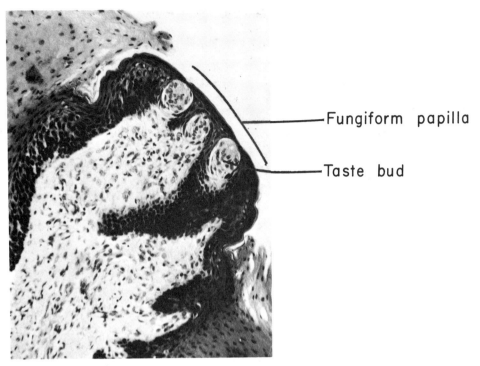

—Fungiform papilla

—Taste bud

Tongue

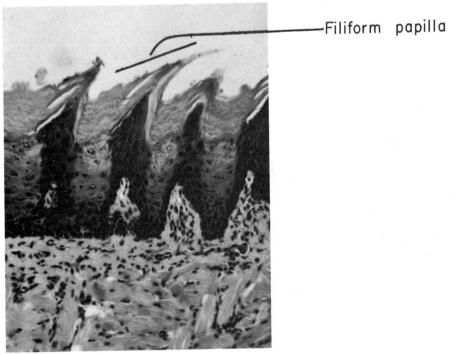

—Filiform papilla

Tongue

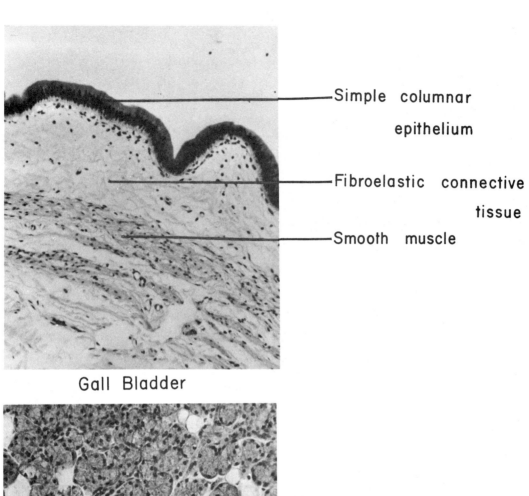

Simple columnar epithelium

Fibroelastic connective tissue

Smooth muscle

Gall Bladder

Fat cell

Serous cells

Parotid Gland

99

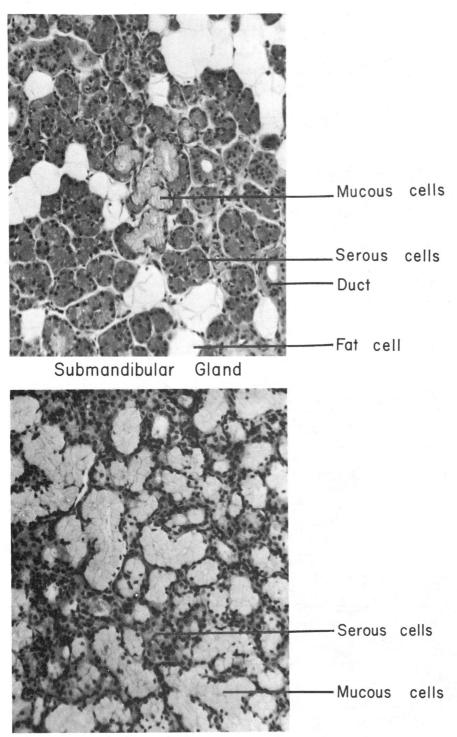

Mucous cells

Serous cells
Duct

Fat cell

Submandibular Gland

Serous cells

Mucous cells

Sublingual Gland

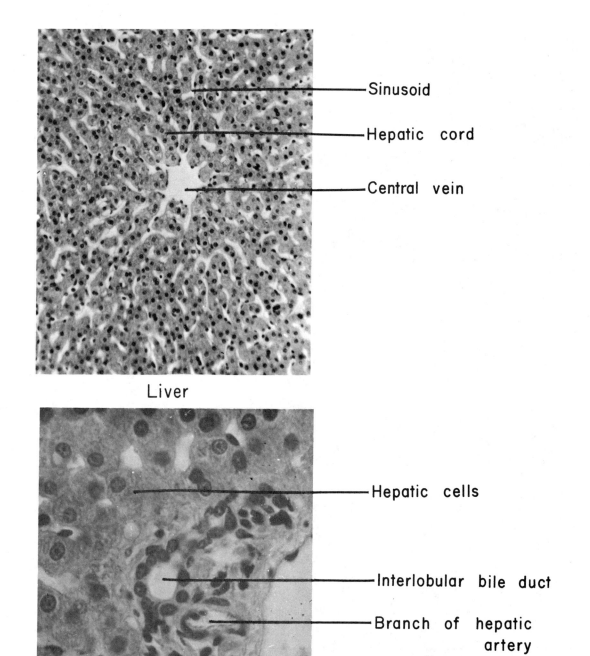

Sinusoid

Hepatic cord

Central vein

Liver

Hepatic cells

Interlobular bile duct

Branch of hepatic artery

Branch of portal vein

Hepatic Triad

101

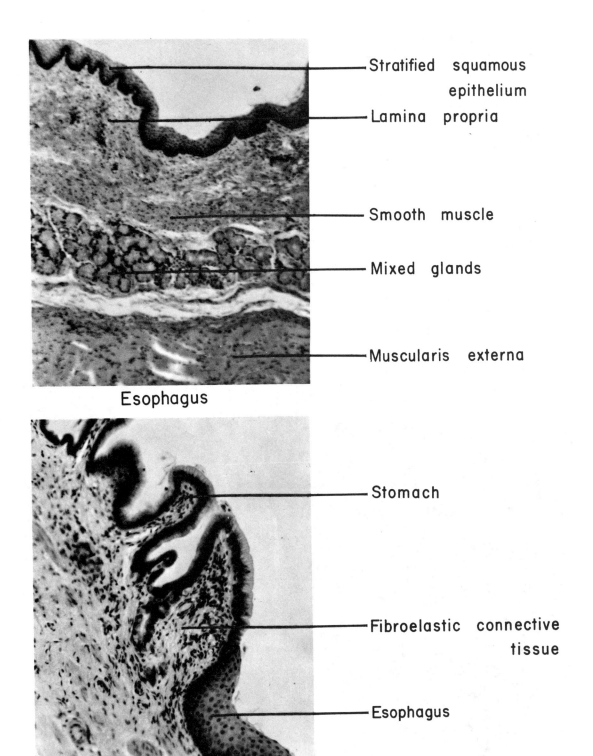

Esophagus

Esophageal-Cardiac Junction

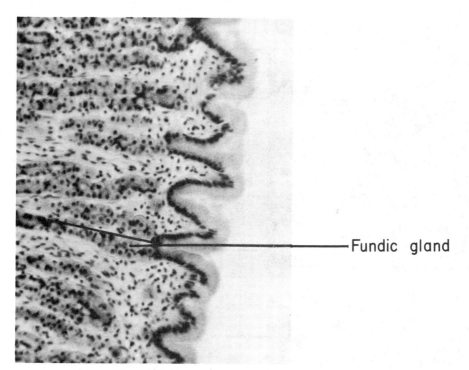

Fundic gland

Fundic Stomach

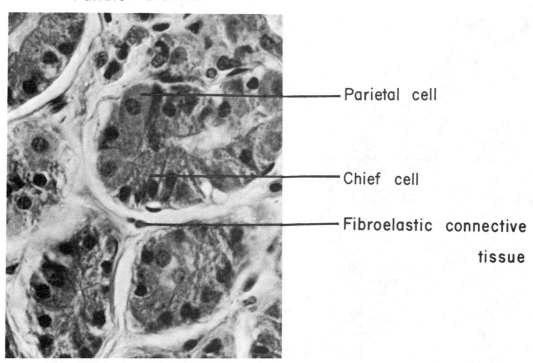

Parietal cell

Chief cell

Fibroelastic connective

tissue

Fundic Stomach

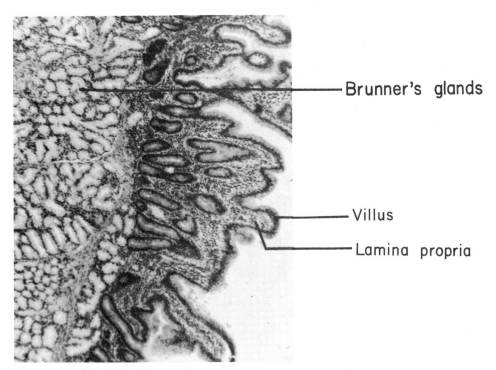

—Brunner's glands

—Villus

—Lamina propria

Small Intestine

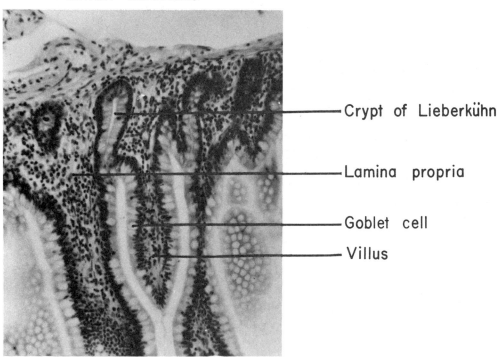

—Crypt of Lieberkühn

—Lamina propria

—Goblet cell

—Villus

Small Intestine

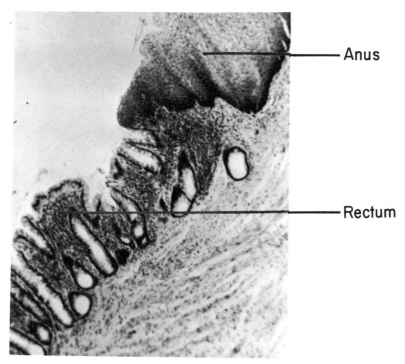

— Anus

— Rectum

Recto-Anal Junction

XIV. THE RESPIRATORY SYSTEM

I. NOSE

A. Nasal cavities

1. Right and left divided by a septum
2. Rigid wall of bone and cartilage
3. Anterior nares (*to exterior*)
4. Posterior nares (*to nasopharynx*)
5. Vestibule (*widest part behind anterior nares*)
6. Respiratory portion (*remainder*)
7. Anterior vestibule: Skin extends into this region containing sebaceous glands, sweat glands, and hair follicles.
8. Respiratory portion: The epithelium becomes pseudostratified ciliated columnar with goblet cells.
9. Mucous membrane: composed of respiratory epithelium, basement membrane, lamina propria (*containing venous sinuses with smooth muscle in walls, FECT, mucous glands, serous glands, lymphatic tissue*) which blends with periosteum or perichondrium in wall of nasal cavity in which case the membrane is called mucoperiosteum or mucoperichondrium, or the Schneiderian membrane.
10. Covers the conchae (*turbinates*).
11. Mucus covers the surface of the respiratory epithelium.

II. ORGAN OF SMELL

A. Olfactory mucosa

1. In the nasal cavity roof extending down over the superior concha.
2. Pseudostratified columnar epithelium, lacking goblet cells, no distinct basement membrane, and three types of cells present.
   a. Sustentacular (*supporting*) cells with pigment granules.
   b. Basal cells with pigment granules.
   c. Olfactory (*bipolar and sensory*) cells with olfactory vesicles and olfactory hairs.
3. Lamina propria (*contains fila olfactoria, lymph plexuses, and serous glands*).

III. PARANASAL SINUSES

A. These are air-filled cavities within the bones of the skull, and are connected with the nasal cavities:

1. Maxillary, frontal, ethmoid, and sphenoid
2. Each sinus is lined by pseudostratified columnar epithelium, goblet cells are less, and the basement membrane not as thick as in nasal cavity.

IV. PHARYNX

    A. Nasopharynx

        1. Is located behind the posterior nares
        2. Mucosa
            a. Respiratory epithelium (*except in regions subject to attrition*)
            b. Lamina propria contains FECT, mostly mucous glands, some serous and mixed glands, and lymphatic tissue.
        3. Submucosa
            a. Laterally, there is loose CT.

    B. Oropharynx

        1. Located behind the oral cavity and posterior surface of tongue.

V. LARYNX

    A. Is a short tubular structure connecting the pharynx and trachea, whose walls contain hyaline and elastic cartilages, FECT, striated muscle, mucous membrane, pseudostratified ciliated columnar epithelium, and mucous and serous glands.

    B. Hyaline cartilage

        1. Thyroid, cricoid, and arytenoid

    C. Elastic cartilage

        1. Corniculates, cuneiforms, and tips of arytenoids; also in epiglottis.

    D. The cartilages and the hyoid bone are connected by three large flat membranes composed of dense FECT.

        1. Thyrohyoid
        2. Quadrate
        3. Cricovocal

    E. False vocal folds: these form the superior border of the laryngeal ventricular aperture.

    F. True vocal folds: these form the inferior border of the laryngeal ventricular aperture.

    G. Mucosa

        1. Above vocal folds is respiratory epithelium.

    2. False vocal fold is covered by respiratory epithelium, and true vocal fold is covered by stratified squamous epithelium.
    3. Below vocal folds is respiratory epithelium.
    4. Epiglottis: anterior and posterior surfaces are stratified squamous epithelium, base is respiratory epithelium.
    5. Lamina propria contains FECT with many elastic fibers, mixed sero-mucous glands, and lymphatic tissue. True vocal folds: prominent elastic fibers, no glands.

H. Submucosa lacking

I. Each vocal fold encloses a vocal ligament, and is bordered laterally by a vocalis muscle.

VI. TRACHEA

A. Mucosa

    1. Respiratory epithelium on a thick basement membrane.
    2. Lamina propria contains delicate FECT and lymphatic tissue bordering the submucosa.

B. Submucosa (*containing many sero-mucous glands*).

C. Adventitia

    1. Contains horse-shoe shaped hyaline cartilages interconnected by FECT. The opening has FECT, a mucous membrane and circular smooth muscle. Mixed glands may penetrate the adventitia, and capillaries are prominent.

VII. LUNG

A. Extrapulmonary bronchi

    1. Resemble trachea in structure, but smaller in diameter.

B. Intrapulmonary bronchi

    1. Appear spherical with no posterior flattening, irregular plates of hyaline cartilage which may encircle the lumen.
    2. Mucosa
       a. Is similar to the trachea, and extrapulmonary bronchi although mucosal folds may be prominent due to contraction of smooth muscle, and has prominent elastic fibers.
    3. Submucosa
       a. Internal to cartilage and is of loose CT with lymphatic tissue (*blends imperceptably with lamina propria*), mixed glands and mucous glands.

4. Adventitia
   a. Cartilage plates are surrounded by dense FECT.

C. Generalization: as bronchi become smaller there is a decrease in
   height of epithelium, a decrease in cartilage and glands, and an
   increase in proportion of elastic fibers and smooth muscle.

D. Bronchioles

1. Usually less than 1 mm in diameter, little or no CT, ciliated
   columnar epithelium with some goblet cells which reduce (*ca.*
   0.3 mm D) to ciliated cuboidal with no goblet cells.
2. Lamina propria: many elastic fibers.
3. Reduction of cartilage and glands.
4. Adventitia: remains as thin CT.
5. The smallest branch is a terminal bronchiole which branches to
   form two or more respiratory bronchioles.

E. Respiratory bronchioles

1. These are ca. 0.5 mm D or less.
2. The epithelium is simple cuboidal or low columnar with cilia
   only in the larger tubes; no goblet cells. External to the
   epithelium the wall is of smooth muscle lying in FECT. A few
   aveoli may outpocket through wall deficiencies. The respiratory bronchioles branch to form 2 to 11 alveolar ducts.

F. Alveolar ducts

1. These are cone-shaped with squamous epithelium lining and a
   wall of FECT with smooth muscle.

G. Alveolar sacs (*open*)

1. Each sac is composed of numerous alveoli.

H. Alveoli (*continuous lining of squamous epithelial cells*) which
   are separated by an interalveolar septum.

I. Interalveolar septum

1. It has a framework of FECT reticular and elastic fibers in
   which are embedded cells.
2. Capillaries and venules for oxygen and carbon dioxide exchange.
3. Cells present within septum:
   a. Endothelial cells of capillary.
   b. Alveolar epithelial cells: small, type A (I) cells and
      large, type B (II) cells. The B cells contain cytosomes
      which produce surfactant.
   c. Macrophages ("dust" cells).
   d. RBC, leukocytes, mast cells, and plasma cells.

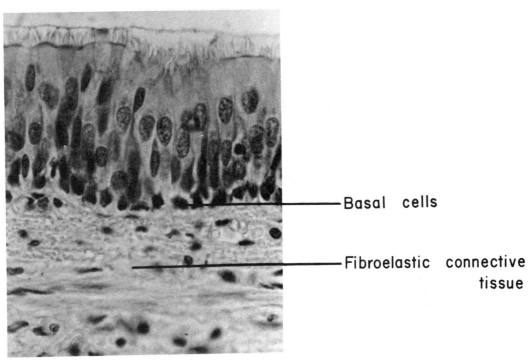

—Basal cells

—Fibroelastic connective
tissue

Pseudostratified Ciliated Columnar Epithelium

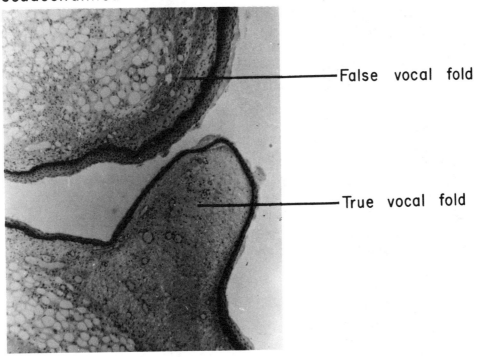

—False vocal fold

—True vocal fold

Larynx

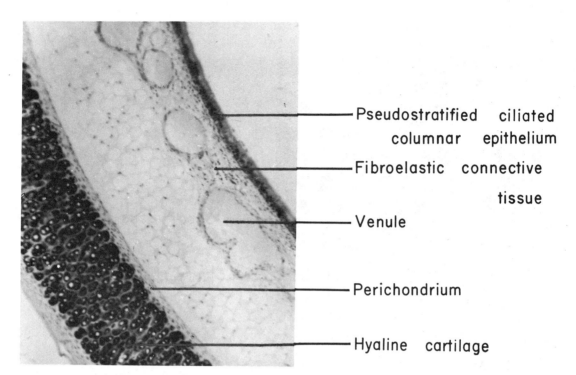

Pseudostratified ciliated columnar epithelium

Fibroelastic connective tissue

Venule

Perichondrium

Hyaline cartilage

Trachea

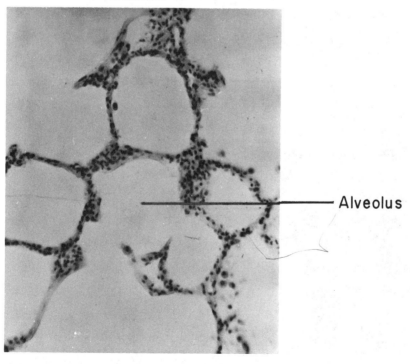

Alveolus

Lung

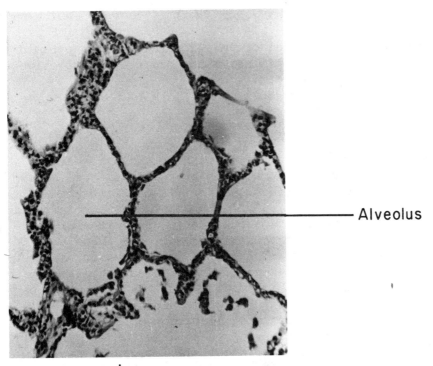

Alveolus

Lung

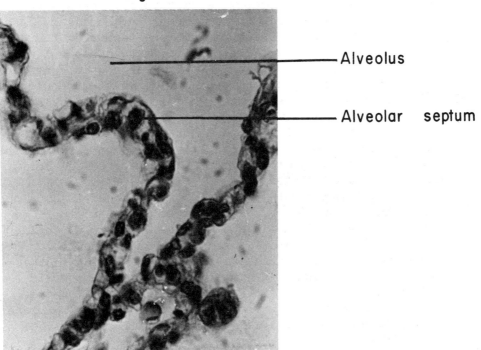

Alveolus

Alveolar   septum

Lung

XV.   THE URINARY SYSTEM

I.   KIDNEY

   A.   Capsule, cortex, medulla, renal columns (*cortex*), renal pyramids
        (*medulla*), medullary rays, papillae, minor calyces, major calyces,
        pelvis, hilum, and blood vessels.

   B.   Nephron - functional unit of kidney

        1.   Renal corpuscle
             a.   Glomerulus: afferent arteriole enters and efferent
                  arteriole leaves at vascular pole; tortuous capillaries
                  of the glomerulus; afferent arteriole has large lumen,
                  lacks a true adventitia, has a thick media whose circular
                  smooth muscle cells at vascular pole are epitheloid-like,
                  pale-staining, with cytoplasmic granules - these are
                  termed "juxtaglomerular" cells which may secrete a hyper-
                  tensive factor called renin. The efferent arteriole has
                  a smaller lumen and thick media which by contraction can
                  regulate pressure within the glomerulus.
             b.   Bowman's capsule: cupshaped dilatation of the nephron
                  with a slit-like capsular space separating the parietal
                  (*outer*) and viseral (*inner*) cell layers.
                  (1)   parietal layer: simple squamous epithelium
                  (2)   visceral layer: podocytes with foot processes called
                        pedicels which lie on the glomerular capillary base-
                        ment membrane. Basement membrane separates pedicels
                        from endothelial cells of capillary. Endothelium is
                        incomplete, with pores. Bowman's space is continuous
                        with the lumen of the proximal convoluted tubule.
             c.   Filtration barrier: separates the blood in glomerular
                  capillaries from the filtrate in the capsular space -
                  (1)   fenestrated, attenuated endothelium
                  (2)   basement membrane (*which also covers entire nephron*)
                  (3)   pedicels of podocytes of visceral epithelial cells
        2.   Proximal convoluted tubule
             a.   Begins at urinary pole of renal corpuscle and is continu-
                  ous with Loop of Henle. The squamous cells of the
                  parietal layer of Bowman's capsule are directly continuous
                  with the simple cuboidal epithelium of the proximal convo-
                  luted tubule. The cells are truncated pyramids, large,
                  pale-staining spherical nuclei, abundant eosinophilic
                  cytoplasm with basal striations (*mitochondria*), and a
                  luminal brush border (*microvilli*); the basement membrane
                  invaginated; lateral plasma membranes seldom observed.
        3.   Loop of Henle
             a.   Replacing the pyramidal, brush-bordered cells of the
                  proximal convoluted tubules are flat, squamous cells which
                  form the descending thin segment of the loop which con-
                  tinues around the loop into the ascending thick segment;
                  cuboidal cells make up the thick segment which ascends to

112

reach the glomerulus and become continuous with the distal convoluted tubule at the vascular pole. The cells of the ascending thick segment have no brush border, more eosinophilic cytoplasm and more basal vertical striations. At the junction the cells adjacent to the afferent arteriole form a disclike region of tall cells, the macula densa.

    4. Distal convoluted tubule
       a. The cells are smaller than those of the proximal convoluted tubule, cuboidal, larger lumen than proximal, and no apparent brush border with LM, and their cytoplasm is less eosinophilic. The distal convolution drains into a collecting tubule which has a different embryological origin than the nephron.

C. Collecting tubule (*excretory ducts*)

    1. Several collecting tubules join to form a
       a. Papillary duct (*of Bellini*) which opens on the surface of a
       b. Papilla which, as a result of the surface openings, appears like a sieve, from which the urine flows to the pelvis.
    2. Tubule cells vary from cuboidal in small tubules to high columnar in papillary ducts; they have a light eosinophilic cytoplasm, and a distinct cellular outline.

D. Blood supply

    1. Abdominal aorta, renal artery (*hilum*) divides into three main branches, interlobar artery (*ascends in a renal column*), arcuate artery (*at corticomedullary junction*), interlobular artery between medullary rays, afferent glomerular arteriole, capillaries, efferent arteriole, stellate veins (*venules*), interlobular vein, arcuate vein, interlobar vein, renal vein, and inferior vena cava.

II. EXCRETORY PASSAGES

A. Pelvis, ureter, and urinary bladder.

    1. Pelvis, in hilum, splits into major and minor calyces; each minor calyx fits cuplike about a medullary papilla; the calyx-pelvis region is an expansion of the ureter.
    2. Mucosa
       a. Transitional epithelium
       b. Basement membrane (EM)
       c. Lamina propria of FECT; some loose, lymphoid tissue; few smooth muscle cells and capillary plexus.
    3. Submucosa not clearly demarcated.

    4. Muscularis
        a. Pelvis: the smooth muscle layers are not clearly demarcated.
        b. Ureter: inner longitudinal and an outer circular coat; the
            lower third of the ureter has a third external longitudinal
            coat.
        c. Urinary bladder: the layers of smooth muscle are not clear-
            ly demarcated, but tend to be inner oblique, middle circu-
            lar, and outer longitudinal.
    5. Adventitia
        a. FECT external to the muscularis. Superior surface of the
            bladder is covered by a serosa.

B. Male urethra

    1. Prostatic urethra
        a. Mucosa: lined with transitional epithelium, and
        b. Lamina propria: highly vascularized (*veins*), abundant
            elastic tissue.
        c. Submucosa: not discernible from the lamina propria.
        d. Muscularis: layers are not well defined.
        e. Adventitia: not well defined.
    2. Membraneous urethra
        a. Lined with tall pseudostratified columnar cells but epi-
            thelium is variable; extends through the urogenital
            diaphram and receives from it some striated muscle cells
            which form the external sphincter of bladder.
    3. Cavernous urethra
        a. Lined with pseudostratified epithelium with patches of
            stratified squamous - variable epithelium.
    4. Glands
        a. Lacunae of Morgagni are invaginations of the mucous
            membrane which may contain single or groups of intra-
            epithelial mucous cells.
        b. Glands of Littré, which are branced tubular, open into the
            lacunae of Morgagni.

C. Female urethra

    1. Mucosa
        a. Lined primarily with stratified, or pseudostratified colum-
            nar epithelium with intraepithelial nests of mucous glands;
            the lamina propria is highly vascularized with veins, abun-
            dant elastic tissue.
    2. Submucosa
        a. Not discernible
    3. Muscularis
        a. Inner longitudinal and outer circular smooth muscle cells,
            but not well defined.
    4. Adventitia
        a. Not discernible.

115

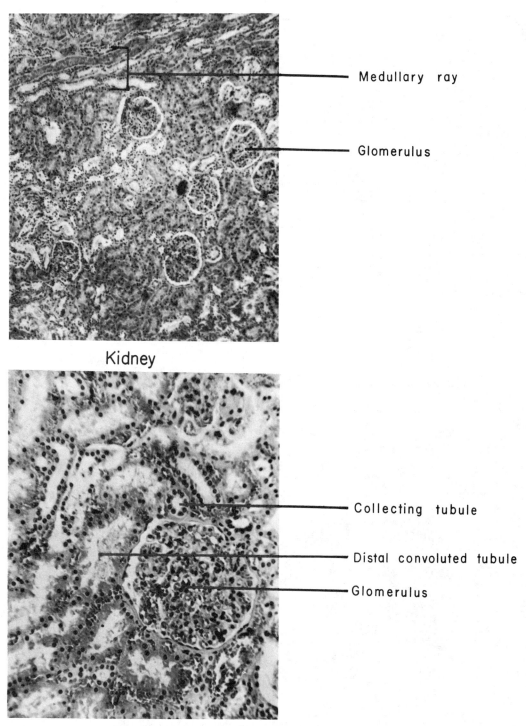

Medullary ray

Glomerulus

Kidney

Collecting tubule

Distal convoluted tubule

Glomerulus

Kidney

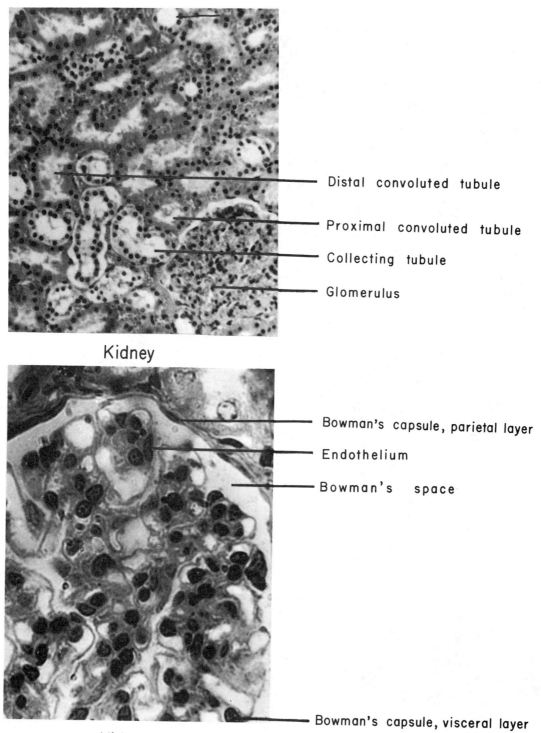

Distal convoluted tubule

Proximal convoluted tubule

Collecting tubule

Glomerulus

Kidney

Bowman's capsule, parietal layer

Endothelium

Bowman's space

Bowman's capsule, visceral layer

Kidney

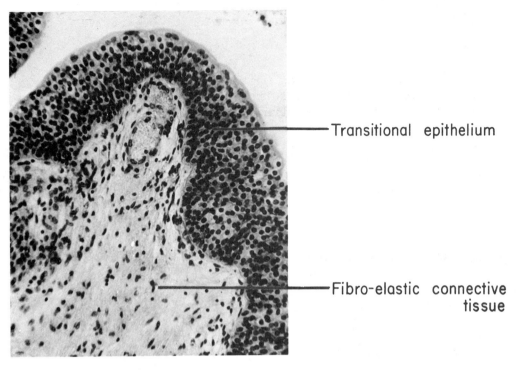

Transitional epithelium

Fibro-elastic connective tissue

Ureter

XVI. THE ENDOCRINE SYSTEM

I. GENERAL CHARACTERISTICS

   A. Ductless glands

      1. Highly vascularized glands which have lost their epithelial
         connection; hormones are secreted directly into the vascular
         system. Parenchyma and stroma are easily identified.
         a. Hypophysis
         b. Thyroid
         c. Parathyroid
         d. Suprarenals
         e. Pineal gland

   B. Mixed glands

      1. Appear as scattered masses in exocrine glands.
         a. Islets of Langerhans - pancreas
         b. Cells of Leydig - testis
         c. Corpora lutea - ovary
         d. Hepatic cells - liver

   C. Structure of glands

      1. Cells appear as clumps, cords, or plates separated by capil-
         laries or sinusoids, and are supported by delicate CT.

   D. Embryonic derivation

      1. Ectoderm
         a. Hypophysis
         b. Suprarenal, medulla
         c. Chromaffin bodies
      2. Mesoderm
         a. Ovary
         b. Testis
         c. Placenta
         d. Suprarenal cortex
      3. Endoderm
         a. Thyroid parenchymal cells
         b. Parathyroid parenchymal cells
         c. Islets of Langerhans

II. HYPOPHYSIS (*PITUITARY GLAND*)

   A. General

      1. The glandular portion is the adenohypophysis which is derived
         from the oral ectoderm - Rathke's pouch. Migrates from oral
         area to definitive position in sella turcica. Neurohypophysis
         is formed as a ventral evagination from the floor of the

forebrain (*diencephalon*). It is covered by an extension of the dura mater, the diaphragma sellae. The hypophyseal stalk passes through an opening in the diaphragm. The gland weighs about 0.5 gm. and is about 1 x 1 x 0.5 cm.

2. Adenohypophysis
   a. Pars distalis
   b. Pars tuberalis
   c. Pars intermedia
3. Neurohypophysis
   a. Pars nervosa (*infundibular process*) lies posterior to the pars intermedia.
   b. Infundibular stem is continuous with the pars nervosa.
   c. Median eminence (*of the tuber cinereum*) is continuous with the infundibular stem.
4. Infundibular (*neural*) stalk
   a. Infundibular stem
   b. Medial eminence

B. Adenohypophysis - pars distalis

1. Surrounded by a fibrous CT capsule, and constitutes about 75% of the hypophysis.
2. Parenchyma is formed by cell cords and cell masses supported by reticular fibers continuous with capsule fibers. Sinusoidal capillaries lie between parencymal cells.
3. Parencymal cells
   a. Chromophils
      (1) acidophils (*35%*) are larger than chromophobes, but smaller than basophils; have eosinophilic granules; they can be separated with differential stains as orangeophils (*alpha acidophils*) using orange G; or carminophils (*epsilon acidophils*) by azocarmine.
      (2) basophils (*15%*) are PAS positive with fewer and smaller granules than acidophils, and are poorly stained by hematoxylin.
   b. Chromophobes (*50%*)
      (1) chief or C cells which have little affinity for dyes, usually no granules in scanty cytoplasm.
4. Hormones
   a. STH (*somatotrophic hormone*) - from acidophils
      (1) somatotrophin stimulates general body growth, especially the epiphyses of bone
         (a) oversecretion - gigantism
         (b) undersecretion - dwarfism
         (c) acromegaly - oversecretion after closing of epiphyseal discs
   b. LTH (*lactogenic hormone or luteotrophic hormone*) - from acidophils
      (1) prolactin promotes mammary gland development and lactation. Maintains corpus luteum and progesterone secretion.

  c. TSH (*thyroid stimulating hormone*) - from basophils.
   (1) thyrotropin stimulates and maintains the thyroid epithelium and general body metabolism.
  d. ACTH (*adrenocorticotropic hormone*) - questionable cellular acidophils
   (1) adrenocorticotropin stimulates the adrenal cortex to secrete cortisol: but has little or no effect on aldosterone.
  e. FSH (*follicle stimulating hormone*) - from basophils
   (1) a gonadotropin which stimulates growth of ovarian follicles in the female, and the testes to produce spermatozoa in the male
  f. (LH)(*luteinizing hormone*) - from basophils
   (1) a gonadotropin converts a ruptured follicle to corpus luteum; ovulation; estrogen secretion
  g. ICSH (*interstitial cell-stimulating hormone*) - from basophils (*same hormone as LH*)
   (1) a gonadotropin (*male luteinizing hormone*) which stimulates the Leydig cells to produce androgen (*testosterone*).
  h. Polypeptide hormones (*acidophils*) - STH, LTH, ACTH
  i. Mucoid hormones (*basophils*) - TSH, FSH, LH
  j. Hypothalamic releasing factors

C. Adenohypophysis - pars intermedia

 1. Is rudimentary and forms about 2% of the hypophysis.
 2. It is composed of a thin layer of cells which may be small, pale staining, and undifferentiated; or larger granular, basophil cells. These basophil cells may extend into the pars nervosa.
 3. It also contains vesicles filled with colloid. Cells lining the vesicles are ciliated.
 4. Secretes MSH (*melanocyte stimulating hormone, a polypeptide*)

D. Adenohypophysis - pars tuberalis

 1. The cells appear as short cords or in clusters aligned closely with blood vessels.
 2. Cells are cuboidal; contains fine cytoplasmic granules, and weakly basophilic; also undifferentiated cells.
 3. Nests of squamous cells may be found around the pars tuberalis.

E. Neurohypophysis

 1. The pars nervosa (*infundibular process*), infundibular stem, and the median eminence of the tuber cinereum all have the same characteristic cells, nerve and blood supply, and contain the same active hormonal principle.
 2. The hypothalamohypophyseal tract containing some 10^5 unmyelinated nerve fibers which pass into the neurohypophysis. The

cell bodies lie in the supraoptic and paraventricular nuclei
of the hypothalamus.
3. Cells
    a. Pituicytes
        (1) resemble neuroglia cells in the CNS, and are abundant
             in the pars nervosa. The cells are small with short
             branching processes ending at blood vessels or CT
             septa. Cytoplasm contains fat droplets, granules,
             and pigment. Four types are identified by silver
             staining:
             (a) reticulopituicytes
             (b) micropituicytes
             (c) fibropotuicytes
             (d) adenopituicytes
4. Granules
    a. Neurosecretory substance elaborated by nerve cells of the
        supraoptic and paraventricular nuclei passes along the
        unmyelinated nerve fibers to the neurohypophysis where it
        is stored.
    b. Neurosecretory substance accumulates in the nerve terminals
        and is called Herring bodies. It stains deeply with chrome
        alum hematoxylin, and is abundant in the pars nervosa
        where it is seen as granules of varying size.
    c. Neurosecretory substance is believed to be associated with
        two hormones of the neurohypophysis.
        (1) vasopressin (*ADH = antidiuretic hormone*) which aids
             in the regulation of water resorption in renal
             tubules; it also causes contraction of smooth muscle
             in blood vessels resulting in a rise of blood pres-
             sure.
        (2) oxytocin which causes a contraction of the smooth
             muscle of the uterus, and also a contraction of the
             myoepithelial (*basket*) cells of the alveoli and ducts
             of the mammary gland.

III. THYROID

   A. Morphology

      1. Thyroid is composed of two lateral lobes connected by an
          isthmus, lying over the 2nd and 4th tracheal cartilages,
          often a median pyramidal lobe.
      2. Outer CT capsule is continuous with deep cervical fascia.
      3. Inner CT capsule extends as septa into gland. Fibroblasts,
          lymphocytes, macrophages, and mast cells occur in the stroma
      4. The lobules are composed of follicles which are embedded in
          fine reticular fibers supporting numerous capillaries.
      5. A follicle consists of a single layer of simple epithelium
          surrounding the contained colloid which may be eosinophilic
          or basophilic.

6. Two kinds of epithelial cells are present on a basement membrane:
    a. Light parafollicular cells that are sparse, not in contact with the lumen, do not contain colloid droplets, and show no polarity; may produce thyrocalcitonin.
    b. Follicular cells which border on the lumen, contain colloid droplets, have a nucleus at the base of the cell; terminal bars as well as microvilli appear on the luminal border.

B. Function

1. Colloid contains enzymes and a glycoprotein called thyroglobulin. It contains diiodothyronine, triiodothyronine, and tetraiodothyronine (*thyroxine*).
2. Thyroxine increases cell metabolism; its release is stimulated by thyrotropin (TSH).

IV. PARATHYROIDS

A. Morphology

1. Variable in number (*2 to 6*) and position. Usually located at superior and inferior poles of thyroid gland; inferior pair are variable. Each gland is a brownish ovoid body about 2 x 3 x 7 mm. weighing about 35 mg; covered by a thin FECT capsule which separates it from the thyroid gland. Fine trabecular extend from the capsule into the gland. Sheets or cords of epithelial cells comprise the parenchyma. The septa carry blood vessels and some nerve fibers.
2. Epithelial cells are of two types:
    a. Chief (*or principal*) cells
        (1) clear cells have a pale staining, agranular cytoplasm with large vesicular nuclei.
        (2) dark cells have smaller nuclei and a fine granular cytoplasm.
    b. Oxyphil cells
        (1) less numerous than chief cells, but are larger with small dark nuclei, and a fine granular eosinophilic cytoplasm.

B. Function

1. Chief cells elaborate the parathyroid hormone which maintains the blood calcium at a nearly constant level, necessary for normal neuromuscular activity.

V. SUPRARENALS

  A. General

    1. Each suprarenal (*adrenal*) gland is a flattened, pyramidal
        shaped cap on the superior pole of the kidney.
    2. An artery enters and a vein exits at the hilum.
    3. Each gland is surrounded by a CT capsule in which two layers
        exhibit; an outer coat of dense fibrous CT, and an inner layer
        of areolar CT containing capillaries. Blood vessels pass into
        the gland, and
        a. Empty into sinusoids of cortex, or
        b. Directly to the medulla
    4. The cortex region develops from mesothelium lining the coelom.
    5. The medulla region develops from primitive autonomic ganglion
        (*sympathochromaffin*) tissue.

  B. Cortex

    1. Zona glomerulosa
        a. Composed of columnar-cuboidal cells in ovoid groups with
            small nuclei and cytoplasm containing lipid droplets.
    2. Zona fasciculata
        a. Parenchyma is composed of cuboidal cells arranged in long
            cords usually two cells wide. Sinusoids separate column
            of cells. The nucleus is vesicular, cytoplasm is basophilic
            and has many lipid droplets which dissolve away in prepara-
            tion leaving the cell with a spongy appearance; hence, they
            are termed spongiocytes.
    3. Zona reticularis
        a. The cell cords form an anastomosing network. Cells are
            usually small, and appear light or dark, depending upon
            presence or absence of pigment granules.

  C. Medulla

    1. Cells are ovoid and occur in groups, or short anastomosing
        cords, surrounded by venules and capillaries.
    2. The cell has a large, vesicular nucleus and a granular cyto-
        plasm. They are called chromaffin cells because the secretory
        cytoplasmic granules appear brown when they are oxidized by
        potassium bichromate. Ganglion cells also present.

  D. Suprarenal function

    1. The cortex is essential to life. It maintains water and
        electrolyte balance, carbohydrate balance, and intercellular
        substances of CT with two distinctive steroid hormones:
        a. Aldosterone promotes the retention mainly of sodium ions
            and excretion of potassium ions. Water may be also retained

as a consequence of sodium retention. Aldosterone has a
hypertensive effect if there is a high level of plasma
sodium. It is secreted primarily by the cells of the zona
glomerulosa.
   b. Cortisol is secreted mainly by the cells of the zona
fasciculata under stimulation by ACTH. Cortisol facili-
tates protein catabolism and gluconeogenesis. It has an
anti-inflammatory factor.
2. The medulla is not essential for life. It produces the
catecholamines - epinephrine and norepinephrine - whose cytoplasmic granule presence can be detected by the chromaffin
reaction. Produced by two separate cell types,
   a. Epinephrine (*adrenalin*) increases oxygen consumption,
mobilizes glucose from liver glycogen, and increases
cardiac output.
   b. Norepinephrine is the mediator of adrenergic nerve impulses
acting on heart and blood vessels to maintain blood pressure.

VI. PINEAL GLAND (*EPIPHYSIS CEREBRI*)

  A. Structure

    1. Is attached to the roof of the third ventricle by a stalk.
    2. It is covered by a capsule formed by the pia mater. Trabeculae
extend inwardly from the pia dividing the body into irregular
lobules. A rich capillary network traverses the septa.
    3. The lobules are composed of two cell types:
     a. Parenchymal (*or chief*) cells or pinealocytes.
      (1) These large clear cells are most numerous. They have
vesicular nuclei, with prominent nucleoli, and a
cytoplasmic basophilia often with lipid droplets.
The slender cytoplasmic processes have bulbous
endings.
     b. Interstitial cells (neuroglia; astrocytes and microglia
are stellate, and the nucleus, cytoplasm and granules
appear more dense than in parenchymal cells.
    4. Calcareous granules (*brain sand*) are concretions usually
present which vary greatly in size and number.

125

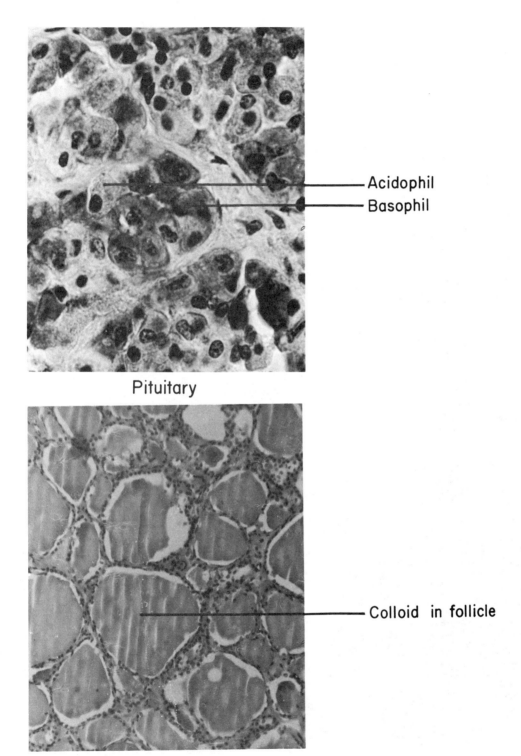

Acidophil
Basophil

Pituitary

Colloid in follicle

Thyroid

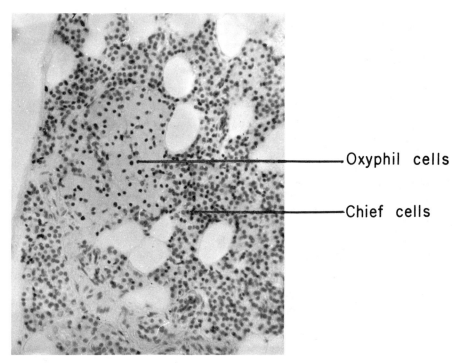

Oxyphil cells

Chief cells

Parathyroid

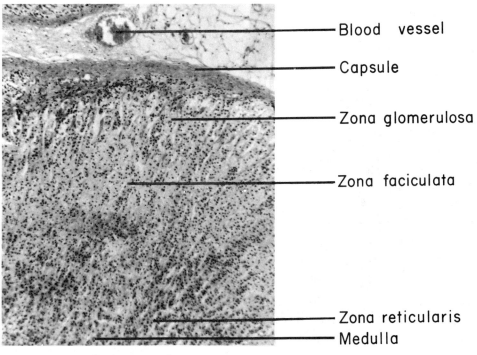

Blood vessel

Capsule

Zona glomerulosa

Zona faciculata

Zona reticularis

Medulla

Suprarenal

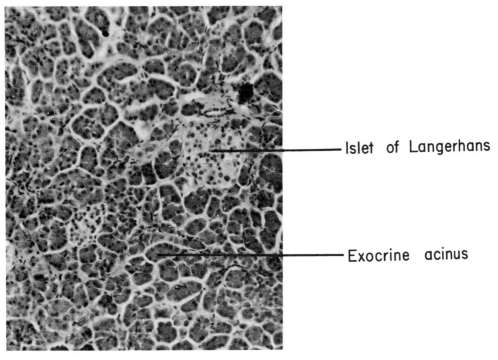

Islet of Langerhans

Exocrine acinus

Pancreas

XVII. THE REPRODUCTIVE SYSTEM

I. MALE REPRODUCTIVE SYSTEM

   A. The testis

      1. Tunica vaginalis
         a. A layer of mesothelium which surrounds the testis lying in the scrotum.
      2. Tunica albuginea
         a. A thick white capsule of dense FECT beneath the t. vaginalis.
      3. Mediastinum testis
         a. A projection of the t. albuginea into the testis along its posterior and superior borders.
      4. Tunica vasculosa
         a. Inner zone of the t. albuginea, very vascular.
      5. Septula testis
         a. Thin fibrous partitions radiating from the mediastinum testis to the capsule which divides the testis into the lobuli testis.
      6. Lobuli testis
         a. Pyramidal compartments with each apex directed toward the mediastinum.
      7. Seminiferous tubules
         a. 1 to 4 convoluted tubules lie in a lobule embedded in loose CT containing vessels, nerves, different types of cells including endocrine.
         b. Interstitial cells
            (1) cells of Leydig
         c. Structure
            (1) germinal epithelium which is a stratified epithelium that lies on a basement membrane. Two types of epithelial cells are
               (a) supporting cells of Sertoli
               (b) spermatogonia
         d. Cells of Sertoli
            (1) tall columnar cells with bases resting on basement membrane.
            (2) nucleus is pale and ovoid.
            (3) prominent nucleolus distinguishes them from spermatogonia cells.
            (4) immature germ cells (*spermatids*) may attach to Sertoli cells.
         e. Spermatogonia
            (1) review "Spermatogenesis".
            (2) review "Spermiogenesis".
      8. Interstitial tissue
         a. Lies between seminiferous tubules containing blood vessels, lymph vessels, nerves, fibroblasts, mast cells, macrophages, and undifferentiated mesenchymal cells as well as cells of Leydig, the interstitial cells which arise from

fibroblasts. These are large cells with vacuoles and pigment in their cytoplasm, and the cells usually occur in groups. There is a prominent nucleolus. Testosterone, produced by the interstitial cells, controls the secondary sex characteristics, the sex impulse, and the development and maintenance of the genital ducts and the accessory glands.

B. The genital ducts

1. Tubuli recti
    a. The seminiferous tubules join at the apex of each lobule to form these straight tubules. Sertoli cells only remain to form a simple columnar-cuboidal epithelium.
2. Rete testis
    a. Straight tubules course to the mediastinum testis to join anastomosing, irregular spaces (*channels*), the rete testis. These channels have a simple cuboidal epithelium resting on a basement membrane. Some cells may bear cilia.
3. Ductuli efferentes
    a. These efferent ductules pass from the mediastinum to connect the rete with the epididymis. CT and smooth muscle cells surround each ductule which is lined by simple columnar cells lying on a basement membrane. Tall columnar cell groups alternate with short cell groups giving lumen an irregular bore. Each cell type may bear cilia, the only motile cilia in the entire duct system.
4. Ductus epididymis
    a. Efferent ductules connect into a single ductus epididymis. It is tortuous, and surrounded by CT. It has a pseudostratified columnar epithelium with basal, and tall columnar cells which may bear stereocilia. The cells rest on a basement membrane which is surrounded by smooth muscle cells. ·
5. Ductus deferens
    a. The coiled ductus epididymis straightens and junctions with the ductus deferens which is present in the palpable spermatic cord.
    b. Mucosa
        (1) pseudostratified columnar epithelium (*tall cells may have stereocilia*) resting on a basement membrane.
        (2) lamina propria contains elastic fibers.
    c. Submucosa
        (1) vascular, CT.
    d. Muscularis externa
        (1) inner longitudinal smooth muscle layer.
        (2) middle circular layer.
        (3) outer longitudinal layer.
    e. Adventitia
        (1) fibrous.

6. Ampulla of ductus deferens - muscle layer less distinct -
   a. Is the terminal dilation which joins the seminal vesicle to form the ejaculatory duct.
7. Ejaculatory duct
   a. Passes through the prostate gland to open into the urethra on a thickened part of the urethral mucosa called the colliculus seminalis. The duct is lined by simple columnar or pseudostratified columnar epithelium.

C. The genital glands

1. Seminal vesicles
   a. Each vesicle is diverticulum off the ductus deferens at the ampulla, long and tortuous.
   b. Mucosa
      (1) pseudostratified or simple columnar epithelial cells which contain secretory pigment granules. Mucosal folds are pronounced. Arcades.
   c. Muscularis
      (1) irregular bundles of smooth muscle
   d. Adventitia
      (1) contains many elastic fibers.
2. Prostate
   a. It surrounds the urethra at its origin from the urinary bladder. It is an aggregate of small compound tubulo-alveolar glands which drain into the prostatic urethra.
   b. The whole gland has a capsule of FECT which contains a plexus of veins. The epithelium is folded and varies from cuboidal to columnar type cells containing secretory granules and lipid droplets. Stroma is dense FECT with smooth muscle.
3. Bulbourethral
   a. Glands of Cowper lie behind the membranous urethra. Each gland is compound tubulo-alveolar, and is surrounded by CT capsule from which septa pass to divide the gland into lobules. CT septa contains elastic fibers, skeletal and smooth muscle cells.
   b. Epithelium is either cuboidal or columnar with mucous droplets.

D. The penis

1. Corpora cavernosa penis
   a. Paired dorsal cylinders of erectile tissue, each surrounded by a FECT sheath (*tunica albuginea*), and skin.
2. Corporus cavernosa urethrae
   a. The single corpus spongiosum is a ventral erectile tissue cylinder containing the cavernous part of the urethra (*See "Urinary System"*). The t. albuginea also surrounds the corpus spongiosum. Composed of venous spaces with FECT between.

E. The seminal fluid

    1. Semen
        a. Seminal fluid is produced by all of the genital glands
            and ducts.
        b. It is whitish and opaque, containing about 6 x 10^4/ ml
            spermatozoa in an ejaculate averaging about 3.5 ml.
        c. Sequence of fluid discharge:
            (1) bulbourethral glands and glands of Littré secrete
                 mucous during erection to lubricate the cavernous
                 urethra.
            (2) prostate discharges first in ejaculation followed by
                 the spermatozoa from the ductus epididymus and ductus
                 deferens.
            (3) seminal vesicles discharge a thick secretion contain-
                 ing fructose.

II. FEMALE REPRODUCTIVE SYSTEM

  A. The ovary

    1. General
        a. Each ovary is attached at its hilum by the mesovarium
            (*peritoneal fold*) to the broad ligament. The free sur-
            face of the ovary is covered by a simple cuboidal epi-
            thelium, often referred to as germinal epithelium. No
            basement membrane is present, but there is dense CT
            (*tunica albuginea*) beneath the epithelium.
        b. Medulla
            (1) inner portion which merges with the vascular loose
                 CT of the mesovarium. It consists of loose FECT
                 with blood vessels, nerves, and smooth muscle cells.
        c. Cortex
            (1) the outer portion is a cellular compact stroma with
                 reticular fibers and spindle-shaped cells resembling
                 smooth muscle cells. Follicles are present in various
                 stages of development. Composed primarily of atretic
                 follicles.
    2. Follicles
        a. Immature ovum surrounded by epithelial cells.
        b. Zona pellucida
            (1) membrane surrounding the ovum.
        c. Liquor folliculi
            (1) a clear fluid contained in spaces in the follicular
                 cell-mass which fuse to form the antrum.
        d. Antrum
        e. Cumulus oophorus
            (1) cell-mass projection into the antrum containing the
                 ovum surrounded by follicular cells.

      f. Corona radiata
        (1) radially arranged follicular cells lying next to the zona pellucida.
      g. Membrana granulosa
        (1) stratified epithelial follicular cells around the antral cavity.
      h. Theca folliculi
        (1) are stroma cells (*sheath*) separated from the membrana granulosa by a basement membrane (*glassy membrane*). CT differentiates into
          (a) theca interna: loose delicate CT containing capillaries and
          (b) theca externa: closely packed collagenous fibers and fusiform cells which merge with surrounding stroma of the cortex.

3. Oogenesis
  a. Review the maturation of the ovum.
4. Ovulation
  a. The mature ovum is discharged at the stigma into the peritoneal cavity and then into the fenestrated end of the fallopian tube.
5. Corpus hemorrhagicum
  a. A newly ruptured follicle with clotted blood which is phagocytized by leucocytes, and invaded by differentiating granulosa cells to form the corpus luteum.
6. Corpus luteum
  a. Granulosa lutein cells are surrounded by theca lutein cells formed by the theca interna. The corpus luteum produces progesterone and estrogen.
7. Corpus albicans
  a. A white scar of CT forms after the corpus luteum degenerates.

B. The fallopian tube

1. Regions
  a. Infundibulum (*with fimbriae*)
  b. Ampulla
  c. Isthmus
  d. Intramural (*portion in uterine wall*).
2. Structure
  a. Mucosa
    (1) simple columnar epithelium some of which are ciliated, no definite basement membrane by light microscopy.
    (2) lamina propria is a cellular CT with scattered smooth muscle cells. Variations occur during the menstrual cycle.
  b. Muscularis externa
    (1) broad inner circular layer of smooth muscle.

             (2) thin outer longitudinal layer.

      c. Serosa

C. The uterus

    1. Regions
        a. Body (*corpus uteri*)
        b. Neck (*cervix*)
        c. Portio vaginalis
        d. Fundus
        e. Isthmus
    2. Structure
        a. Perimetrium
            (1) typical serosa
        b. Myometrium
            (1) muscularis externa
                (a) stratum subvasculare (*inner longitudinal layer*).
                (b) stratum vasculare (*middle circular vascular layer*).
                (c) stratum supravasculare (*outer longitudinal layer*).
        c. Endometrium
            (1) mucosa
                (a) simple columnar epithelium with scattered groups of ciliated cells.
                (b) uterine glands extend through the mucosa in the stroma of the lamina propria. Stroma is composed of stellate cells, leukocytes and blood vessels.
                (c) cystic changes result in an obstruction of the gland.
            (2) proliferative (*follicular*) stage, with endometrial changes.
            (3) progestational (*secretory*) stage, with endometrial changes.
            (4) ischemic (*premenstrual*) stage, with endometrial changes.
            (5) menstrual stage, with endometrial changes.
    3. Uterus in pregnancy
        a. Blastocyst
            (1) embryo (*inner cell mass*).
            (2) trophoblast (*outer cell layer*).
                (a) cytotrophoblast (*inner cell layer*).
                (b) syncytial trophoblast (*outer cell layer*).
                     (1) primary villi.
                     (2) secondary (*chorionic*) villi.
                (c) chorion frondosum.
                (d) chorionic plate.
                (e) chorion laeve.

              b. Decidua
                  (1) capsularis
                  (2) basalis
                  (3) parietalis
              c. Lacunae
          4. Cervix
              a. Mucosa - doesn't participate in menstruation.
                  (1) tall, simple columnar epithelial cells which secrete
                       mucus; some are ciliated.
                  (2) lamina propria is a cellular CT containing large
                       glands.
                  (3) in the vaginal portion, the epithelium is moist,
                       stratified squamous.
              b. Muscularis externa
                  (1) smooth muscle bundles appear in dense collagenous CT.

      D. The vagina
          1. Structure
              a. Mucosa
                  (1) thick, nonkeratinized stratified squamous epithelium.
                       Cytoplasm contains much glycogen.
                  (2) lamina propria has elastic fibers, lymphocytes, and
                       often lymph nodes.
              b. Muscularis externa
                  (1) inner circular smooth muscle layer is thin.
                  (2) outer longitudinal layer is thick.
              c. Adventitia

      E. The external sex organs

          1. Clitoris
              a. Rudimentary, consists of two cavernous erectile bodies,
                  and is covered with stratified squamous epithelium.
          2. Labia minora
              a. Form lateral walls of the vestibule. These mucous mem-
                  brane folds have a stratified squamous epithelium and a
                  core of vascular CT. Sebaceous glands appear on each sur-
                  face of the fold.
          3. Labia majora
              a. Folds of skin covering the labia minora. Inner surface is
                  smooth, and the outer surface has a cornified epidermis
                  with hairs, sweat and sebaceous glands, and adipose tissue.
          4. Vestibule
              a. The vagina and urethra open here. It is lined with strati-
                  fied squamous epithelium, and contains minor vestibular
                  glands about the urethral opening. In the lateral walls
                  are the major vestibular glands, analagous to the bulbour-
                  ethral glands in the male.

F. The mammary gland

1. General
    a. A modified sweat gland with apocrine secretion, located
        within the subcutaneous tissue.
    b. The gland consists of 15 to 20 lobes. Each lobe is an
        individual gland with its own lactiferous duct opening
        at the nipple area.
    c. Fat and CT surround each lobe, and divide each lobe into
        lobules.
2. Areola and nipple
    a. Areola
        (1) pigmental epidermis area extending peripherally
             around the nipple which contains glands (of Mont-
             gomery). Sweat and sebaceous glands as well as
             hairs are present.
    b. Nipple
        (1) skin is pigmented.
        (2) dermis contains tall papillae and smooth muscle cells.
        (3) lactiferous ducts open on the surface.
3. Inactive gland
    a. Intralobular ducts are narrow.
    b. Myoepithelial basket cells lie between the epithelium and
        the basement membrane.
    c. Alveoli appear as buds off ducts.
    d. CT between lobes is abundant, dense and coarse.
4. Active gland
    a. Secretory ducts become enlarged and extended, and fat dis-
        appears during the first half of pregnancy. Later, alveoli
        become enlarged, and the lobes become distinct entities.
        Decrease of fat and FECT; increase of glandular material.
    b. During lactation, the alveoli are prominent and closely
        packed. Epithelium of alveoli varies from simple cuboidal
        with lipid material at apical end to simple squamous
        (after discharge of secretion). There is apocrine type of
        secretion. Intralobular ducts are similar to alveoli in
        structure and function.
    c. After lactation, milk in the alveoli lumina is absorbed,
        and regressive changes occur to return the gland to the
        resting state.

136

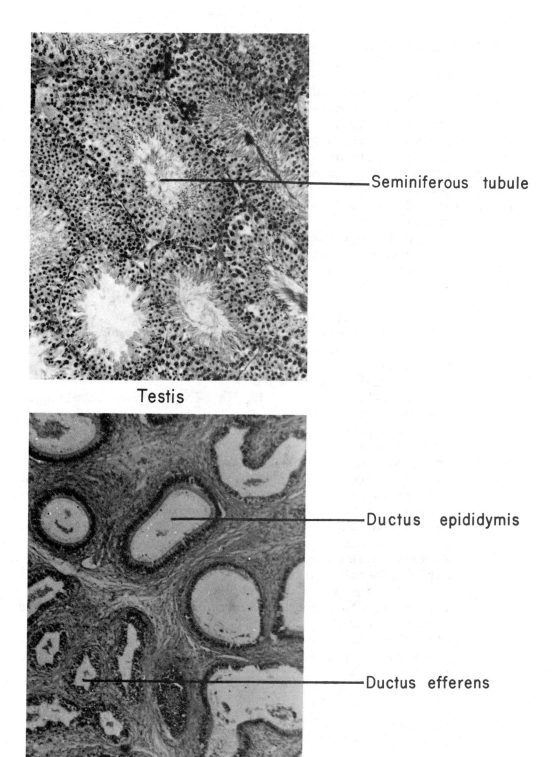

Seminiferous tubule

Testis

Ductus epididymis

Ductus efferens

Mediastianum Testis

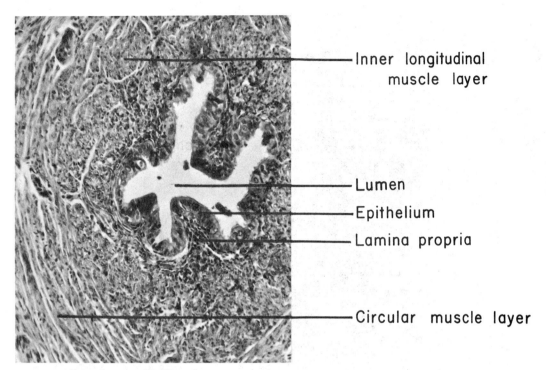

Inner longitudinal
muscle layer

Lumen

Epithelium

Lamina propria

Circular muscle layer

Ductus Deferens

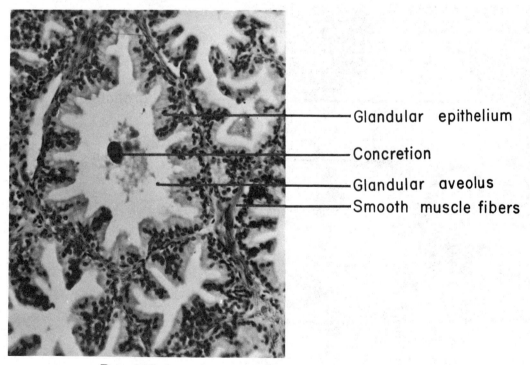

Glandular epithelium

Concretion

Glandular aveolus
Smooth muscle fibers

Prostate

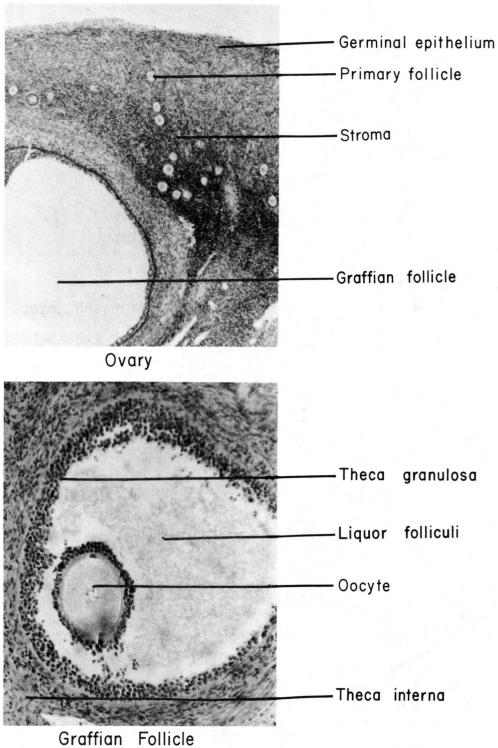

Germinal epithelium

Primary follicle

Stroma

Graffian follicle

Ovary

Theca granulosa

Liquor folliculi

Oocyte

Theca interna

Graffian Follicle

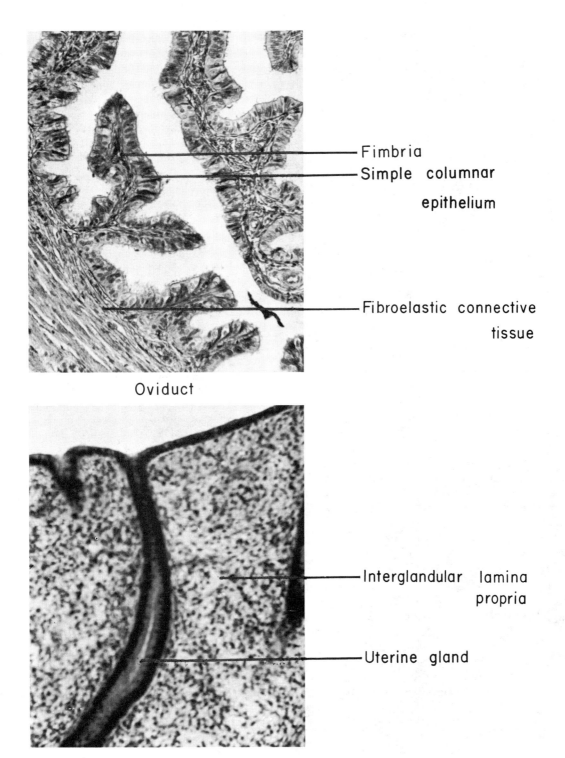

Fimbria

Simple columnar
epithelium

Fibroelastic connective
tissue

Oviduct

Interglandular lamina
propria

Uterine gland

Uterus

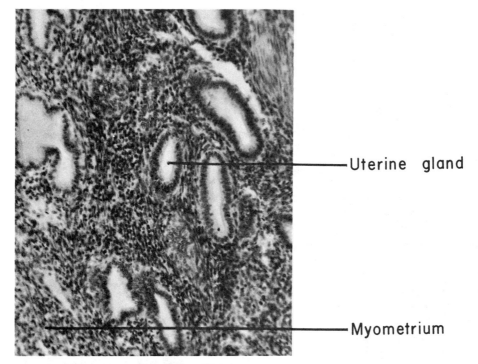

Uterine gland

Myometrium

Uterus - Proliferative

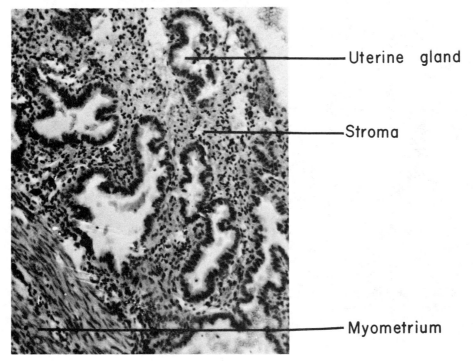

Uterine gland

Stroma

Myometrium

Uterus - Secretory

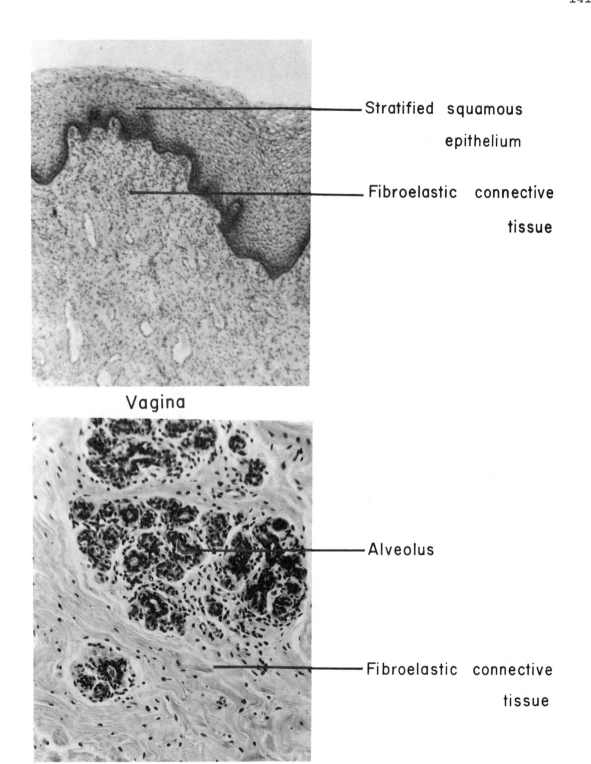

Stratified squamous epithelium

Fibroelastic connective tissue

Vagina

Alveolus

Fibroelastic connective tissue

Mammary Gland

XVIII. THE EYE

I. FIBROUS TUNIC

A. Sclera

1. Episcleral layer
    a. A mixture of loosely arranged collagen and elastic
        fibers which is very vascular. This layer attaches
        anteriorly the lining of the eyelid (*conjunctiva*) to the
        sclera.
2. Sclera proper
    a. Made up of interlacing collagen fibers and few elastic
        fibers serving for tendon attachment of the extrinsic
        muscles of the eye; also fibroblasts.
3. Lamina fusca
    a. It contains pigment cells and many elastic fibers.
4. Lamina cribrosa
    a. The perforated disk of the sclera through which the fibers
        of the optic nerve pass posteriorly.
    b. The scleral walls are continuous with the dural, arachnoid,
        and pial sheaths of the optic nerve.

B. Cornea

1. Corneal epithelium
    a. Stratified squamous epithelium with free nerve endings.
        Minor injuries heal rapidly.
2. Bowman's membrane
    a. A randomly arranged network of collagenous fibrils.
3. Corneal stroma (*substantia propria*)
    a. Makes up about 90% of cornea with collagenous fibers ar-
        ranged in thin lamellae. Also contains fibroblasts,
        lymphoid wandering cells, fine elastic network, chondroitin
        sulfate, and keratosulfate.
4. Descemet's membrane
    a. Elastic basement membrane for (*probably*) the
5. Corneal mesenchymal epithelium
    a. A single layer of large squamous cells covering inner
        surface of Descemet's membrane.

II. VASCULAR TUNIC (UVEA)

A. Choroid

1. Extends anterior to the ora serrata of the retina.
2. Suprachoroid
    a. Consists of loose CT in a series of thin slanting
        lamellae. Each membranous lamella contains melanoblasts,
        fibroblasts, and elastic fibers, some smooth muscles, and
        no blood vessels.
3. Vessel layer

        a. Contains many medium and large arteries and veins with
            loose CT between them along with collagenous fibers and
            stellate pigment cells.
    4. Capillary layer
        a. One of wide-bored capillary network with a stroma of col-
            lagenous and elastic fibrils, and some fibroblasts.
    5. Glassy membrane (*Bruch's*)
        a. Non-cellular composed of two lamella.
           (1) outer; elastic fibrillae
           (2) inner; cuticular
           (3) in part, the basement membrane of the pigment layer
               of the retina.

B. Ciliary body

    1. This part extends from the ora serrata anteriorly to the
        scleral spur, and is the anterior extension of both retina and
        choroid.
    2. Ciliary processes.
    3. Ciliary muscle.
    4. The suspensory ligament of the lens is attached to the ciliary
        body at the zonula.

C. Iris
    1. It is a thin membranous structure which is a continuation of
        the ciliary body. Its posterior surface rests on the anterior
        surface of the lens. It also divides the anterior from the
        posterior chambers which are filled with lymphlike aqueous
        humor.
    2. Layers
        a. Endothelium covers anterior surface.
        b. Anterior border layer determines color of iris by chromato-
            phores.
        c. Vessels, delicate collagenous fibrillae have some elastic
            fibers and chromatophores.
        d. Dilatator pupillae and sphincter pupillae smooth muscles
            control pupil size.
        e. Pigment epithelium is densely pigmented layer on posterior
            surface and reflects light.
    3. Iris angle
        a. Formed at the lateral borders of the anterior chamber, and
            is composed of loose CT forming a meshwork containing the
            spaces of Fontana. The meshwork and Schlemm's canal form
            a means of exit from the eye of the aqueous humor. It is
            apparently formed by secretory activity of the ciliary
            epithelium of the ciliary processes. The humor circulates
            from the posterior to the anterior chamber of the eye. If
            proper drain-off (*venous*) does not occur at the iris angle,
            an increase in intraocular pressure results in glaucoma.

III. INNER TUNIC

    A. Retina

        1. Inner portion (*neuronal links are underlined*)
            a. Internal limiting membrane is a thin homogeneous membrane
                formed by the expanded ends of the radical fibers of
                Muller's.
            b. Nerve fiber layer
                (1) contains axons of ganglion cells (*these axons con-
                     verge at the optic disk, acquire a myelin sheath,
                     and form the optic nerve*), neuroglia cells, blood
                     vessels and inner branches of Müller's fibers.
            c. Ganglion cell layer
                (1) consists of a single layer of typical *multipolar
                     ganglion cells* and some neuroglia cells together
                     with some blood vessels.
            d. Inner plexiform layer
                (1) this consists of the axonic processes of amacrine
                     cells, and the axons of the bipolar cells which
                     synapse with the dendrites of the ganglion cells.
            e. Inner nuclear layer
                (1) herein lie the nuclei of the *bipolar cells*, horizontal
                     cells, amacrine cells, and of Müller's supporting
                     fibers. Blood vessels from the inner retina extend
                     into this layer.
            f. Outer plexiform layer
                (1) a reticular meshwork in which the axons of the rods
                     and cones synapse with the dendrites of the bipolar
                     cells.
            g. Outer nuclear layer
                (1) formed by the closely packed nuclei of the *photore-
                     ceptors*.
            h. External limiting membrane
                (1) a sievelike membrane composed by the chief supporting
                     elements of the retina called Müller's fibers.
            i. Rods and cones layer
                (1) consists of dendritic cytoplasmic processes of the
                     photoreceptors packed side by side.
        2. Outer portion
            a. Pigment epithelium layer
                (1) developed from the outer ectodermal layer of optic
                     cup.
                (2) single layer of cells, cuboidal or hexagonal, with
                     pigment called fuscin, intimate with the cuticular
                     lamella of choroid and loosely attached to the rest
                     of retina.

IV. MACULA LUTEA AND FOVEA CENTRALIS

   A. Fovea centralis is a posterior pole depression of the visual axis
       with closely packed cone cells. The macula lutea is the yellow
       region surrounding the fovea. Visual acuity is greater here.

V. ORA SERRATA

   A. The anterior limit of the functional retina.

VI. OPTIC NERVE

   A. The retinal unmyelinated nerve fibers converge at the optic disk
       (*blind spot*), pass through the lamina cribrosa, and form the optic
       nerve. It is actually a fiber tract connecting the retina with
       the brain rather than a peripheral nerve like other cranial nerves.
       It consists of myelinated fiber bundles without neurilemma and is
       ensheathed by the meningeal brain coverings. Glial cells are found
       between the fibers. The middle part is occupied by the central
       artery and vein which reach into the inner nuclear layer of the
       choroid and the nerve fiber layer of the retina.

VII. LENS

   A. Capsule

       1. Structureless, elastic membrane on which the fibers of the
           suspensory ligament insert.
       2. Anterior epithelium is the simple cuboidal cell layer on the
           anterior lens surface. There is no posterior epithelium.
       3. Lens nucleus
           a. Lens fibers arranged in concentric lamellae united by an
               amorphous cement substance.
       4. Zonula ciliaris (*suspensory ligament*) connects ciliary body to
           lens.

VIII. VITREOUS BODY

   A. Occupies the space between the lens and retina.

       1. Composition
           a. 99% water
           b. Hyaluronic acid
           c. Vitrein (*protein*)
       2. Patellar fossa
           a. Broad shallow depression on anterior surface.
       3. Hyaloid canal
           a. Site of fetal hyaloid artery coursing from the optic disc
               to the patella fossa.

    4. Hyaloidea
        a. Peripheral condensation of the vitreous.

IX. EYELIDS

    A. Review histology related to the following structures:
        thin skin, conjunctiva, obicularis oculi muscle, superior
        palpebral muscle, tarsal plate, meibomian glands, (*sebaceous*)
        glands of Zeis, (*sweat*) glands of Moll, lacrimal glands, glands
        of Krause, glands of Wolfring.

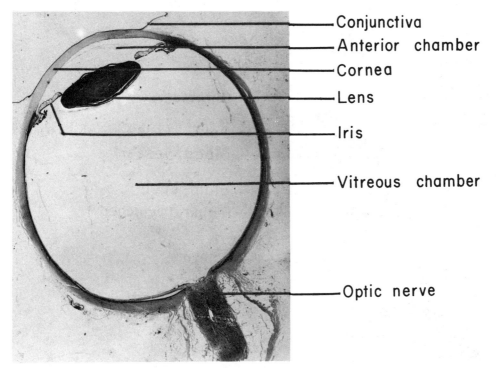

Conjunctiva
Anterior chamber
Cornea
Lens
Iris
Vitreous chamber
Optic nerve

Eye

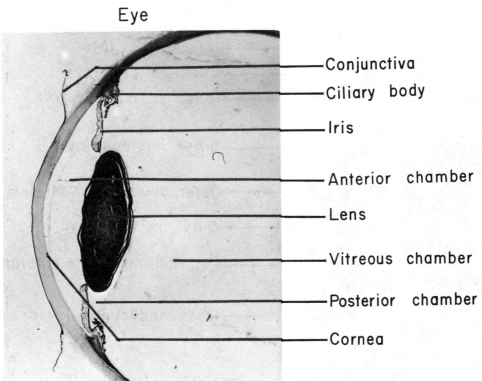

Conjunctiva
Ciliary body
Iris
Anterior chamber
Lens
Vitreous chamber
Posterior chamber
Cornea

Eye

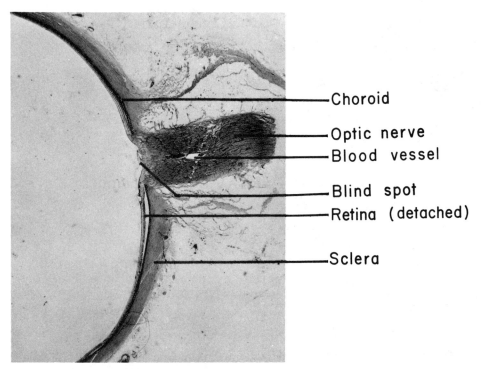

—Choroid

—Optic nerve
—Blood vessel

—Blind spot
—Retina (detached)

—Sclera

Eye

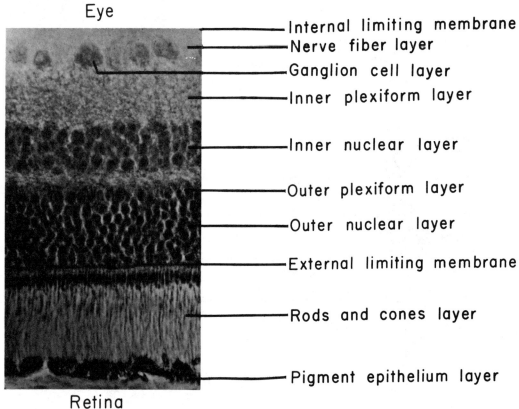

—Internal limiting membrane
—Nerve fiber layer
—Ganglion cell layer
—Inner plexiform layer

—Inner nuclear layer

—Outer plexiform layer

—Outer nuclear layer

—External limiting membrane

—Rods and cones layer

—Pigment epithelium layer

Retina

From Woolff's Anatomy of the Eye and Orbit, 6th edition, Fig. 96, page 100, W.B. Saunders Co., Philadelphia, by R.J. Last.

XIX. THE EAR

I. EXTERNAL EAR

   A. Auricle or pinna

      1. Internal core of elastic cartilage.
      2. Covered by perichonorium and thin skin.
      3. Vestigeal muscles.
      4. Skin contains hairs, few sweat glands, and sebaceous glands.
      5. Lobule contains fat and CT, but no cartilage.

   B. External auditory meatus

      1. Outer 1/3 is supported by elastic cartilage
      2. Inner 2/3 is a canal through the temporal bone
      3. Continuation of auricular skin lines the tube
      4. Sebaceous glands and hairs in cartilagenous part
      5. Skin contains ceruminous glands that are modified sweat glands (*apocrine type*) which contain brown pigment granules and fat droplets.
      6. Cerumen is a brownish, waxy substance formed by the secretions of ceruminous and sebaceous glands, plus desquamated cells.

   C. Tympanic membrane

      1. Thin skin is continuous with that of meatus.
      2. Outer radial collagenous fiber layer and the inner circular collagenous fiber layer. These two regions are lacking in the upper flaccid layer of the membrane.
      3. Inner surface is covered by a mucous membrane of simple squamous cells.

II. MIDDLE EAR

   A. Tympanic cavity

      1. 1/2" x 1/2" cubed air space lined by a mucous membrane. The epithelium is generally simple, squamous and non-ciliated with no basement membrane and a thin lamina propria present. Upon infection, the epithelium may become stratified squamous or ciliated cuboidal.
      2. Auditory bones (*ossicles*)
         a. Malleus - attached to tympanic membrane.
         b. Incus - middle bone.
         c. Stapes - basal plate is fixed to the oval window of the median wall which also contains the round window.
         d. The ossicles have no epiphyses, are full-sized in fetal life, the stapes have (*in adult*) marrow, the ends are

covered by articular cartilage, the malleus and incus are
suspended by ligaments, a mucous membrane wraps around the
ossicles, and the stapes is in direct contact with the
perilymph of the inner ear.

e. Tympanic antrum (*and mastoid cells*) is lined by a mucous
membrane that is continuous with that of the tympanic
cavity.

f. Eustachian tube connects the anterior tympanic cavity to
the nasopharynx and is lined by a mucous membrane. The
upper 1/3 is bony, the mucous membrane is continuous with
that of the tympanic cavity, and the epithelium is simple,
ciliated columnar. The lower 2/3 is cartilage (*upper
hyaline and lower elastic*), the epithelium is pseudostratified columnar and ciliated. Some lymph nodules occur in
the lamina propria and mixed sero-mucous glands in the
submucosa.

g. Muscles - tendons attach to ossicles.
    (1) tensor tympani pulls the malleus inwardly by its
    handle.
    (2) stapedius pulls the stapes outwardly by its neck.

h. Nerves
    (1) V (*trigeminal*) nerve innervates the tensor tympani.
    (2) VII (*facial*) nerve innervates the stapedius muscle.

III. INTERNAL EAR

A. Contained in the petrous part of the temporal bone and is about
2/3" long.

1. Externally - bony labyrinth of canals and chambers which are
the
    a. Semicircular canals
    b. Vestibule
    c. Cochlea
    d. Lining is periosteum with mesenchymal epithelium on the
    free surface and containing a fluid, the perilymph.

2. Internally - membraneous labyrinth of closed tubes and chambers with exterior fibrous CT and lined internally by simple
squamous epithelium. They are surrounded by perilymph and
filled with similar, but separate, fluid - the endolymph.
    a. Those parts related to static kinetic senses: the five
    parts are
        (1-3) 3 semicircular canals, each bearing a swollen
            ampulla at one end, both ends uniting with the ellip-
            soidal
        (4) utricle - which communicates with the sphenoidal
        (5) saccule by a tube from which the endolymphatic duct
            is derived; it terminates in the endolymphatic sac
            under the dura of the posterior part of the temporal
            bone.

b. Vestibule separates the semicircular canals and cochlea
    and is occupied by the saccule and utricle.
c. Those parts related to the auditory sense.
    (1) maculae: thickened sensory areas on utricle and
         saccule of simple squamous epithelium.
         (a) sensory hair cells and VIII nerve
         (b) sustentacular cells.
         (c) otolithic membrane covers surface of macula
              whose upper surface has particles named octoconia
              of CaCO3 and a protein.
    (2) cristae: each ampulla of semicircular duct bears one
         with same structure (cells)of maculae. The cupola is
         comparable to the otolithic membrane, but it lacks
         otoconia. Intimate with vestibular nerve (VIII branch)
         as is the maculae.

B. Bony cochlea

    1. Modiolus - axial pillar
        a. Spiral lamina - projecting shelf
        b. Basilar membrane - extends from free border of spiral
            lamina to outer wall which divides the spiral canal into
            two compartments
    2. Superior - scala vestibuli: one end joins the perilymphatic
        space of the vestibule (oval window) and the apical end joins
        with lower scala through the helicotrema.
    3. Inferior - scala tymphani: both scalae are lined with simple
        mesenchymal epithelium. The scala tymphani lining is contin-
        uous with the secondary tympanic membrane covering the round
        window.

C. Cochlear duct: small membranous tube inside the bony cochlea from
    a blind end to the saccule via the

    1. Ductus reuniens: There is an external covering of fibrous CT
        and internal simple squamous epithelium. The roof is the
    2. Vestibular membrane which separates the perilymph of the scala
        vestibuli from the endolymph of this duct.
    3. Spiral ligament is the lateral surface of the duct and blends
        with the periosteum of the bony cochlea. The thick pseudo-
        stratified epithelium and fibrous CT form the
    4. Stria vascularis that may be the source of endolymph.
    5. Basal surface - floor of duct: it is elevated and specialized
        for hearing as the
    6. Spiral organ of Corti.
        a. Basilar membrane is beneath and lateral to the spiral
            organ. It has about 25,000 collagen-like fibers (auditory
            strings) embedding in a homogeneous ground substance which
            provide a supporting base for

      b. Cells of the spiral organ. From without toward the modiolus these are

        (1) peripheral cells
           (a) cells of Cladius - cuboidal.
           (b) cells of Hensen.
        (2) outer hair cells - columnal.
        (3) outer phalangeal cells (*cells of Deiters*) - columnar cell, one for each hair cell support.
        (4) inner and outer pollar cells - between these is formed the inner tunnel.
        (5) inner phalangeal cells.
        (6) inner hair cells.
        (7) border cells.

D. Tectorial membrane: its lower surface rests on the tips of hairs of the hair cells.

E. Nerves

    1. Auditory nerve (*VIII*)
      a. Vestibular branch.
        (1) supplies maculae.
        (2) supplies cristae.
      b. Cochlear branch (*VIII*)
        (1) supplies the spiral organ of Corti.

GLOSSARY

ACIDIC DYE A neutral salt whose staining property is in the acidic radical; e.g., cytoplasm is acidophilic.

ACIDOPHILS Cells which are susceptible to acid stains, such as those found in anterior hypophysis.

ACINUS A group or cluster of cells. Usually glandular.

ADIPOSE TISSUE Tissue which is composed of a varying number of fat cells.

ADVENTITIA A layer of fibro-elastic connective tissue, usually as an external coat of blood vessels or other organs.

AFFERENT Carrying toward; i.e., fibers which carry impulses toward the central nervous system.

ALBUMIN A simple protein, widely distributed throughout the tissues of plants and animals.

ALVEOLI Thin walled sacs found in the lung. Wall is composed of many capillaries, and diffusion of O_2 and CO_2 occurs here.

AMELOBLASTS Tall columnar cells which form enamel.

ANASTOMOSE Means of intercommunication between two structures; e.g., blood vessels.

ANGSTROM UNIT One ten-millionth of a meter; i.e., one ten-thousandth of a micron. (*Abbreviated Å*).

APOCRINE GLAND A type of secretion by which the apical end of the cell is pinched off and becomes part of the secretory product.

APPENDIX The vermiform process located at the ilio-cecal junction of the intestine.

ARACHNOID The middle membrane covering the brain and spinal cord.

ARGENTAFFIN CELLS Cells which take a silver stain; function is synthesis of 5-hydroxytryptamine.

ARGYROPHILIC Cells or products of cells which have an affinity for silver.

ARTIFACT A structure that has been produced by artificial means. An organ or tissue which has been changed from its natural state.

ATROPHY An acquired reduction in size.

AUERBACH'S MYENTERIC PLEXUS The myenteric plexus situated between the longitudinal and circular layers of muscle concerned with autonomic supply of the gastro-intestinal tract.

AUTOLYSIS Self-destruction of cells or tissue, usually by release of self-contained enzymes.

AUTONOMIC NERVOUS SYSTEM Includes all of the neural apparatus concerned with visceral functions.

ATRIO-VENTRICULAR NODE A portion of the impulse conducting system of the heart found in the subendocardium of the median wall of the right atrium close to the coronary sinus.

AXON A process of a nerve cell that normally conducts away from the cell body.

BASEMENT MEMBRANE A rather homogeneous mass underlying epithelium and composed of reticular fibers and protein polysaccharides (*basal lamina*).

BASIC DYE A neutral salt whose staining property is in the basic radical; e.g., the nucleus is basophilic.

BASOPHILS Cells which have an affinity for basic stains, such as in the anterior hypophysis.

BONE A supportive, rigid connective tissue with a calcified matrix, osteocytes and fibers.

BRUNNER'S GLANDS Submucosal glands of the duodenum which are mucous-secreting.

BRONCHIOLES Tubular structures which connect trachae with alveoli in lung. Walls are usually composed of epithelium, fibroelastic connective tissue, smooth muscle, cartilage, and glands.

BRUSH BORDER (*microvilli*) Projections of plasma membrane at apical end of cell, probably for the function of adding surface and metabolic area to the cell.

CAPILLARY A blood vessel composed of endothelium and a varying amount of supportive connective tissue.

CAPSULE Dense fibro-elastic connective tissue surrounding an organ or structure.

CARDIAC GLANDS One of the branched tubular glands of the stomach. Invaginations of mucosa of the stomach.

CARTILAGE   A rather rigid, supportive form of connective tissue.   Matrix composed of chondrocytes and chondrotin.

CECUM   The first portion of the large intestines.   A pouch-like sac off the ascending colon.

CEMENTUM   Forms a thin sheath on the surface of the dentin of the anatomical root of the tooth.

CENTRIOLE   A minute rod or granule considered to be the active, self-perpetuating, division center of the cell.

CEREBELLUM   The posterior brain mass, lying above the pons and medulla and beneath the posterior portion of the cerebrum; it controls the muscular coordination of the body.

CEREBROSPINAL FLUID   Located in the subarachnoid space (*between pia and arachnoid*) and ventricles, produced by the choroid plexus.

CEREBRUM   The principal portion of the brain, excluding the cranial vault, the medulla, pons and cerebellum.

CHIEF (*zymogenic*) CELLS   Cells of the gastric glands that secrete pepsin. Zymogen granules are found at apical end and RNA at the base of cell.

CHOROID   The vascular tunic of the eye; continuous with the iris in front.

CHROMOPHILS   Cells of the anterior pituitary which are subdivided into acidophils and basophils according to their staining reactions with hematoxylin and eosin.

CHROMAFFIN   Cells which have an affinity for chromium stains; e.g., cells of adrenal medulla.

CHROMATIN   Typical appearance of the elongated chromosomes in the interphase nucleus; the condensed portions of the chromosomes appear densely stained with hematoxylin.   DNA, RNA, histones and nonhistones have been identified in isolated chromatin.

CHROMOPHOBES   Cells of the anterior pituitary which have very little affinity (*or none*) for stains.

CHROMOTROPE   The ratio of dye to substrates.   If insufficient dye is present, metachromasia will not occur.

CILIA   Cytoplasmic projections of a cell, motile, and usually at apical surface.

COLLAGENOUS FIBERS   These are called white fibers in their fresh state. They are composed of collagen and arranged in wavy bundles of fibrils which, in electron micrographs, show a periodicity of 640 Å.

COLLOID A rather homogenous mass of material found within follicles of many glands such as thyroid, pars intermedia of pituitary.

COLON (*Large Intestine*) The division of the large intestine extending from the caecum to the rectum.

CONJUNCTIVA Mucous membrane covering the anterior portion of the globe of the eye and reflected upon the lids.

CORNIFIED The degenerative process by which cells of stratified squamous epithelium are converted into dry, horny, dead plates.

CORPUS ALBICANS A structure found in the ovary, resembling a scar, and produced by the degeneration of a corpus luteum.

CORPUS HEMORRHAGICUM A corpus luteum containing blood, found directly after ovulation.

CORPUS LUTEUM A structure found in the ovary remaining after rupture of the Graafian follicle.

CORTEX Pertains to the superficial zones, layers or area of an organ or structure.

CROSS SECTION A section produced by cutting at a right angle to the longitudinal axis of an organ, tissue, or other structure.

CROWN The part of the tooth that is above the gum margin.

CRYPTS OF LIEBERKÜHN Invaginations of the intestinal mucosa and lined by columnar-cuboidal cells, and goblet cells. Paneth cells are found at base of a crypt (*gland*).

CYTOPLASM The protoplasm of the cell, other than the nucleus. Contains inclusions and cellular organelles; mitochondria, endoplasmic reticulum, Golgi, etc.

DEMILUNE A cluster of glandular cells in which the serous cells are displaced to the blind end of the acinus and "cap" the mucous cells.

DENDRITE One of the branching protoplasmic processes of the nerve cell. Normally conducts toward the cell body.

DENTAL PAPILLA The primordium of the pulp.

DENTIN Forms the bulk of the tooth and gives the main strength to it; composed of collagenous fibers in a calcified ground substance.

DEOXYRIBONUCLEIC ACID (DNA) A polymer of nucleotides whose sugar is desoxyribose. Exists as a polymer anion. Concentrated in the chromatin of the nucleus in helical ladder forms.

DERMIS Corium or true skin composed of white and yellow elastic fibers. Layer of skin between the epidermis and subcutaneous tissue.

DESMOSOME Specialized areas of connection between adjacent cellular membranes (*macula adherens*).

DUODENUM The first portion of the small intestine. Histologically, may be subdivided into two different areas.

DURA MATER The outermost covering of the brain and spinal cord.

DYES Neutral salts having both acidic and basic radicals.

ECTODERM After establishing the primary germ layers, it is the outer layer of cells in the embryo. Epidermis and neural tube, e.g., develop from ectoderm.

EFFERENT Conducting away from the central nervous system.

ELASTIC CARTILAGE Rather flexible cartilage whose matrix contains many elastic fibers. Found in epiglottis and external ear.

ELASTIC FIBERS Fibers found in fibro-elastic connective tissue, very flexible, infractile and composed of elastin. In fresh state, they appear pale yellow.

ENAMEL Material which covers the crown of the tooth.

ENDOCARDIUM A layer lining the interior of the heart, consisting of endothelium and a thin layer of connective tissue.

ENDOCRINE GLAND Ductless glands which produce hormones to regulate many metabolic processes of the body; e.g., pituitary, thyroid, adrenal, etc.

ENDODERM The innermost of the three primary germ layers of the embryo. Forms lining of gut and respiratory system, etc.

ENDOPLASMIC RETICULUM A canalicular system of membranes found within the cytoplasm. (a) Rough endoplasmic reticulum - outer surface studded with ribosomes (RNA). (b) Smooth endoplasmic reticulum - no ribosomes are found on the surface of the membranes.

ENDOTHELIUM Flat cells forming the lining of the blood vessels.

EOSINOPHIL Cells with an affinity for acid stains. One of the leukocytes.

EPENDYMA The membrane lining the central canal of the spinal cord and the cerebral ventricles. Consists of ciliated cuboidal or columnar cells.

EPICARDIUM The visceral layer of pericardium that immediately envelops the heart, consisting of fibro-elastic connective tissue.

EPIDERMIS The outer protective, epithelial layer of skin.

EPIMYSIUM Dense fibro-elastic connective tissue (*sheath*) which surrounds an entire muscle.

EPIPHYSES Refers to the end(s) of bone which ultimately become consolidated with the principal portion of bone.

EPITHELIUM A group of contiguous cells forming a tissue, with a minimum amount of intercellular material. Lines gut, respiratory system, genito-urinary system; forms epidermis.

ERYTHROCYTE A mature red blood corpuscle.

EXOCRINE GLAND A gland which conveys its secretions via a duct system.

FASCIA Regular fibro-elastic connective tissue, usually in sheets.

FASCICULUS A small band or bundle of fibers; usually muscle or nerve fibers.

FENESTRATED Having window-like openings, e.g., elastic plates of the aorta.

FIBER A filamentous, elongated structure.

FIBRINOGEN A globulin of the blood plasma that is converted into coagulated protein, fibrin, by the action of thrombin in the presence of ionized calcium.

FIBROBLAST An elongated flattened cell present in connective tissue.

FIBROELASTIC CARTILAGE Similar to hyaline cartilage but containing an excessive amount of collagen in its intercellular substance; an example is a tendon insertion.

FIBRO-ELASTIC CONNECTIVE TISSUE (FECT, CT) A tissue composed of cells, fibers and ground substance. A supportive tissue.

FOLLICLE A crypt or minute lacuna.

FUNDIC GLANDS Distributed through the greater part of the gastric mucosa.

FUSIFORM Spindle-shaped.

GALL BLADDER A pear-shaped organ lying obliquely on the inferior surface of the liver; it may be regarded as a diverticulum of the bile duct.

GANGLION   An aggregation of nerve cells.

GERMINAL CENTER   An active center producing lymphocytes in lymphatic tissue.

GERMINAL EPITHELIUM   A specialized type of epithelium, found in the ovary and testes, which connotes oogenesis and spermatogenesis.

GINGIVA (*GUM*)   The connective tissue and mucus membrane covering the alveolar ridge and necks of the teeth.

GLAND   A secreting organ.

GLANDS OF LIEBERKÜHN   Simple tubular glands in the mucous membrane of the small intestine.

GLOMERULUS   A tuft of capillary loops found in the kidney, where filtration of plasma and production of urine occurs.

GOBLET CELLS   Unicellular mucous glands of the intestinal and respiratory tracts.

GOLGI COMPLEX   An organelle comprised of three components: vacuoles, aggregations of smooth-surfaced double layered membranes; and micro-vesicles or granules concerned with secretion and packaging of secretory products in a cell.

GRAAFIAN FOLLICLE   A hollow sac found only in mammals containing fluid secreted apparently by lining follicle cells. The fluid covering the ovum projects from a mound of follicle cells.

GRAY MATTER   The central column of the spinal cord composed principally of nerve cells and transversely directed fibers; "H" shaped.

HAIR FOLLICLE   A keratinized structure growing from the skin.

HAVERSIAN SYSTEM   One of Havers' canals with lamellae of bone surrounding it.

HEMOCYTOBLAST   A primitive blood cell derived from embryonic mesenchyme.

H AND E STAIN   Hematoxylin and eosin are commonly used in routine tissue staining to stain nuclei blue and cytoplasm pink.

HILUM   A central depression of an organ or structure with a concentration of connective tissue and usually where arteries enter and veins leave.

HISTOLOGY   Microscopic anatomy named by Owen in 1844.

HOLOCRINE GLAND A gland whereby the entire cell becomes part of the
  secretory product.

HYALINE CARTILAGE The usual form of permanent nonarticular cartilage.

HYPERTROPHY Overgrowth.

HYPOPHYSIS (*pituitary gland*) Endocrine gland. Composed of pars distalis,
  intermedia, nervosa and tuberalis. Produces and secretes tropic hormones.

ILEUM The third part of the small intestine.

INTERCALATED DISK The junction of two cardiac muscle cells.

INTERSTITIAL Relating to spaces.

INTRACARTILAGINOUS BONE FORMATION Bone which forms in cartilage, by first
  eroding the cartilage, then laying down the calcified matrix.

INTRAMEMBRANOUS BONE FORMATION Bone which is formed on a matrix of fibro-
  elastic connective tissue.

ISLETS OF LANGERHANS Groups of cells found in the pancreas, arranged as
  anastomosing cords. Produce and secrete insulin and glucagon. Consist
  of
        alpha cells: glucagon
        beta cells : insulin
        delta cells: unknown function

JEJUNUM The second part of the small intestine.

JUNCTIONAL COMPLEX A typical junctional complex of columnar epithelium:
  zonula occludens (*tight junction*), zonula adherens (*loose junction*), and
  macula adherens (*desmosome*). These zones of membrane fusion may exhibit
  independently in other cells.

KERATIN A scleroprotein present largely in cuticular structures, such as
  the hair.

LACUNA A small depression.

LAMELLA A thin sheet or scale.

LAMINA PROPRIA Delicate, fine, fibro-elastic connective tissue found
  beneath the basement membrane of epithelium, in gastro-intestinal
  system, etc.

LEUKOCYTE Any one of the white blood cells.

LEYDIG CELL (*Interstitial cell of the testis*) Found in the area between seminiferous tubules in the testis; produces testosterone.

LIVER The largest gland of the body lying in the right upper abdominal quadrant.

LOBE One of the subdivisions of an organ.

LOBULE A small lobe or subdivision of a lobe.

LONGITUDINAL SECTION A cut or division made parallel to the long axis of a body.

LUMEN The space in the interior of a tubular structure.

LYMPH NODE A network of lymphatic tissue filtering blood.

LYMPHOCYTES Hematogenous cells, white blood cells; reactive in antigen-antibody reactions.

LYSOSOME Organelles rich in acid phosphatase; (*suicide, autolytic bags of the cell*).

MACROPHAGES (*Histiocyte*) A phagocytic cell found in fibro-elastic connective tissue and reticulo-endothelial system.

MAST CELLS Cells found in connective tissue, contain metachromatic granules, and produce heparin.

MATRIX The ground substance of a cell or tissue.

MATURATION A stage of cell division in the formation of cells.

MEDULLA Refers to the inner (*deeper*) area of an organ, e.g., adrenal medulla which is surrounded by the cortex.

MEISSNER'S PLEXUS A submucosal plexus composed of small ganglia concerned with the autonomic innervation of the gastro-intestinal system.

MEIOSIS A process of cell division in which the chromosome number is reduced from a diploid to a haploid number.

MELANOCYTE (*melanoblast*) The cell responsible for the production of melanin.

MENINGES The membranes that envelop the brain and the spinal cord; dura mater, arachnoid, and pia mater.

MEROCRINE GLAND One whose product is secreted by the cells, the latter not being thereby destroyed.

MESENCHYME   An aggregation of mesenchymal cells derived from the embryo.

MESOTHELIUM   Simple squamous epithelium lining the pleural, pericardial and peritoneal cavities. From mesoderm.

MESODERM   The middle of the three primary germ layers of the embryo.

METACHROMASIA   A staining of a tissue component so that the absorption spectrum of the dye-complex differs from that of the original dye; i.e., there is a change in color.

MICRON   One one-millionth of a meter or one one-thousandth of a millimeter.

MICROVILLI   Submicroscopic projections of cell membrane; brush border, striated border.

MITOCHONDRIA   Cellular organelles containing many enzymes; supplying energy for many cellular chemical reactions. The "power plant" of the cell.

MITOSIS   A process of cell division in which the chromosome number keeps the diploid condition.

MONOCYTE   A relatively large mononuclear leukocyte in the circulating blood.

MUCOPOLYSACCHARIDES (*protein polysaccharides*)   These form the ground substance of connective tissue. They may be sulfated (*chondroitin sulfates and kerotohyalin*) or non-sulfated (*hyaluronic acid and chondroitin*).

MUCOSA   The mucous membrane.

MUCOUS   Relating to mucus of a mucous membrane.

MUCOUS GLANDS   Glands which secrete a mucous product, such as goblet cells, and glands of the gastro-intestinal system.

MUCOUS MEMBRANE   The wet epithelial lining of the digestive tract, and other internal passageways; it consists of 3 layers: an epithelial lining, a supporting lamina propria and a muscularis mucosa.

MUSCULARIS EXTERNA   A muscular layer on external surface of the gastro-intestinal tract composed of smooth and/or skeletal muscle in 2-3 layers.

MUSCULARIS MUCOSA   It is the third and outermost layer of a mucous membrane, consisting generally of two thin layers of smooth muscle fibers together with varying amounts of elastic tissue.

MYELIN SHEATH   A sheath of myelin surrounding the nerve fiber deep to the neurolemma.

MYOCARDIUM The cardiac muscle of the heart.

MYOEPITHELIAL CELL A cell found in a number of organs such as the mammary glands, ducts, which have contractile abilities.

NEPHRON The functional unit of the kidney consisting of glomerulus and tubular system.

NEUROGLIA (*glia*) The interstitial tissue of the nervous system composed of astroglia, oligodendroglia, microglia, and ependyma.

NEUROLEMMA The covering of all nerve fibers of the peripheral nervous system; also known as the sheath of Schwann. The cells are derived from neuro-ectodermal cells.

NEURON (*nerve cell*) The structural unit of the nervous system.

NEUTROPHIL A mature white blood cell in the granulocytic series.

NISSL BODIES Found in the perikaryon and dendrites of nerve cells; the basophil substance (*tigroid bodies*).

NUCLEAR MEMBRANE A double-layered structure from 250 to 400 A thick enveloping the nucleus; inner membrane is smooth while outer is rough as a result of fine RNA granules adhering to its outer surface.

NUCLEOLUS A spherical accummulation of chromatin and RNA found within a nucleus.

NUCLEOPLASM The protoplasm or colloid portion of the nucleus of a cell.

NUCLEUS A differential mass of protoplasm, the coordinating center of the functional activity of a cell.

ODONTOBLAST Peripheral tall columnar cells which form dentin.

ORGAN OF CORTI A specialized complex membranous structure extending the length of the cochlea and is composed of hair cells, the receptors of sound stimuli, and various supporting cells.

ORGANELLE A specialized metabolic part of a cell analogous to an organ.

OSSIFICATION The natural process of bone formation.

OSTEOBLAST A bone-forming cell.

OSTEOCLAST A giant cell with a variable number of nuclei closely associated with areas of bone resorption.

OSTEOCYTE The mature bone cell found in a lacuna.

PACINIAN CORPUSCLE It is an elliptical body composed of concentric layers of connective tissue with a soft core, through which an axon terminates. It is sensitive to deep pressure.

PANCREAS A compound tubulo-acinar gland, posterior to the stomach, secreting digestive enzymes, insulin and glucagon.

PANETH CELLS Cells found mainly in the bottom of crypts of Lieberkühn containing large apical secretory granules.

PARASYMPATHETIC DIVISION The cranio-sacral division of the autonomic nervous system.

PARATHYROID GLAND Rather small glands, found in proximity to the thyroid gland, which secrete parathormone which, in turn, regulates calcium metabolism.

PARENCHYMA The specialized portion of an organ or tissue, as opposed to the supporting tissue, stroma.

PARIETAL CELLS The HCl-secreting cells of the gastric glands, truncated in shape.

PAROTID GLAND A salivary gland located on the masseter muscle inferior and anterior to the ear. Secretion contains digestive enzymes.

PARS NERVOSA Posterior lobe of the pituitary, composed primarily of pituicytes with close association with the hypothalamic-hypophyseal tract.

PARS DISTALIS A portion of the anterior lobe of the pituitary gland, which produces many tropic hormones.

PARS INTERMEDIA A portion of the pituitary gland, composed of follicles, crypts and anastomosing cords of cells, which produces intermidin, a melanocyte stimulating hormone.

PARS TUBERALIS Portion of the pituitary which forms a cuff around the hypophyseal stalk; composed of acidophils, basophils, and undifferentiated cells.

PERICHONDRIUM Dense fibro-elastic connective tissue which surrounds cartilage.

PERIODONTAL MEMBRANE Connective tissue which surrounds the root of the tooth.

PERIOSTEUM Dense fibro-elastic connective tissue which surrounds bone.

PEYER'S PATCHES Lymphoid follicles in the distal portion of the ileum of the small intestines.

PHAGOCYTE A cell possessing the ability to ingest foreign particles or cells harmful to the body.

PIA MATER The innermost membrane covering the brain and spinal cord.

PITUICYTES The parenchymatous cell of the pars nervosa. Usually with long processes and contain pigment.

PLASMA MEMBRANE Cytoplasmic membrane which surrounds the cell.

PROLIFERATION The growth and reproduction of similar cells.

PROTHROMBIN Thromboplastin from the platelets transforms prothrombin into thrombin which transforms fibrinogen into fibrin in the coagulation of blood.

PROTOPLASM Living matter of a cell.

PSEUDOSTRATIFIED CILIATED COLUMNAR (*respiratory epithelium*) Epithelium which is primarily found in the respiratory tract. Each cell touches the basement membrane.

PYLORIC GLANDS Glands of the stomach confined to the pyloric region.

PULP The soft vascular tissue in the central part of the tooth.

PURKINJE FIBERS Modified cardiac muscle conduction cells; contain more sarcoplasm and glycogen.

PYCNOTIC A degenerative change in which the nucleus appears smaller and chromatin is condensed; usually appears darker than normal.

RETICULO-ENDOTHELIAL SYSTEM (RES) A group of different kinds of cells in the body which are phagocytic that form a system of macrophages.

RETINA The light-receptive layer of the eye.

RECTUM The terminal portion of the digestive tube.

REFLEX ARC An arrangement whereby a motor and a sensory neuron are linked together synaptically as a receptor-effector mechanism.

RETE MIRABILE A vascular network interrupting the continuity of an artery or vein.

RIBONUCLEIC ACID A type of nucleic acid concerned with protein synthesis in the cell.

RETICULAR FIBERS Fibers of fibro-elastic connective tissue which take a silver stain (*argyophilic*) and usually are not seen in regular hematoxylin and eosin preparations. Compose stroma of lymphoid organs. Chemically related to collagen.

RIBOSOME An organelle in the cell which is the site of protein synthesis. Composed of RNA and proteins.

ROOT One to three projections of a tooth below the gum margin.

SALIVA A clear, tasteless, odorless, slightly acid viscid fluid.

SARCOMERE The contractile unit of a myofibril bounded by Z disks in striated muscle.

SINO-AURICULAR NODE A division of the specialized conduction system of the heart found in the subendocardium at the junction of the superior vena cava and right atrium.

SCHNEIDERIAN MEMBRANE The mucoperiosteum or mucoperichondrium in the nasal cavities formed by a blending of the mucous membrane with the periosteum or perichondrium, and lining the respiratory portion.

SCHWANN SHEATH Schwann cells which cover a nerve fiber forming the neurolemma.

SCLERA The fibro-elastic connective tissue forming the white of the eye.

SEBACEOUS GLAND Usually associated with the hair follicle; simple or branched alveolar glands which secrete sebum.

SEMINIFEROUS TUBULES Tubular structures found in the testes, containing developing sperm.

SEROSA A serous membrane.

SEROUS GLANDS Glands composed of the cells which have zymogen granules (*protein secretion*) at apical end and prominent RNA at base.

SERTOLI CELLS A columnar cell found in the seminiferous tubules for support and/or nutrition of sperm.

SHARPEY'S FIBERS Connective tissue fibers by which the periosteum is attached to the underlying bone.

SIMPLE COLUMNAR EPITHELIUM Epithelium composed of a single layer of columnar shaped cells. Found in gastro-intestinal system, kidney tubule, etc.

SIMPLE CUBOIDAL EPITHELIUM Epithelium composed of a single layer of cuboidal shaped cells. Found in the thyroid gland, ducts, etc.

SIMPLE SQUAMOUS EPITHELIUM Epithelium composed of a single layer of squamous cells. Found in the kidney tubules, lining blood vessels (*endothelium*) etc.

SINUSOID A large space or channel for the passage of blood; it does not contain the defined coats of an ordinary blood vessel.

SMOOTH MUSCLE Muscle composed of spindle shaped cells. Found in the walls of blood vessels, viscera, and is usually involuntary.

SPERMATIDS Male germ cell just before mature sperm in development.

SPERMATOGONIA Primative male germ cell found at the periphery of the seminiferous tubules.

SPINAL CORD The nervous system can be divided into the central nervous system (*brain and spinal cord*) and the peripheral nervous system (*cranial and spinal nerves with their ganglia*); that portion of the nervous system found in the vertebral column.

STELLATE Star-shaped.

STEREOVILLI (*microvilli*) Protoplasm projections at apical end of cell. Usually non-motile (*stereocilia*).

STRATIFIED SQUAMOUS EPITHELIUM Epithelium composed of many layers of cells.a Surface cells are squamous. May be keratinized as in the skin or non-keratinized as in the esophagus.

STRATUM CORNEUM Thorny dead or dying, superficial layer of the skin.

STRATUM GERMINATIVUM The basal germinative layer of the epidermis. Deepest layer with many mitotic figures. This layer, along with the stratum spinosum, makes up the stratum malpighii.

STRATUM GRANULOSUM The granular layer of the skin. Granules composed of keratohyalin.

STRATUM LUCIDUM The layer of epidermis just beneath the stratum corneum. Homogeneous appearing. Absent in thin skin.

STRATUM SPINOSUM The prickle-cell layer on the basal cell layer of the epidermis.

STRIATED MUSCLE Muscle which is typically composed of transverse bands which may be anisotropic or isotropic. Cardiac muscle is involuntary; skeletal muscle is voluntary.

STROMA The supporting framework of an organ. Usually connective tissue.

SUBLINGUAL GLAND A salivary gland located in the floor of the oral cavity, composed of both mucous and serous cells.

SUBMANDIBULAR GLAND A salivary gland located in the submandibular triangle, primarily composed of serous cells, with a few mucous cells.

SUBMUCOSA Layer of connective tissue found in the gastro-intestinal system connecting epithelium to deeper layers.

SUPRARENAL (*adrenal*) GLAND Endocrine gland found at superior pole of the kidney. Produces hormones which pertain to protein and carbohydrate metabolism, inflammation and mineral metabolism.

SWEAT GLANDS Found over the entire body surface with a few exceptions; they are simple coiled tubular glands.

SYMPATHETIC DIVISION The thoraco-lumbar portion of the autonomic nervous system.

SYNAPSE The area where a nerve impulse is transmitted from one neuron to another.

SYNCYTIUM A multinucleated mass of protoplasm resulting from a fusion of many cells. Example is a skeletal muscle cell.

TENDON Regular, dense fibro-elastic connective tissue composed of collagenous fibers and fibroblasts.

TERMINAL BAR A heavy dark-staining area surrounding the apical cellular surface which includes the tight junction (*zonula occludens*) and the loose junction (zonula adherens).

THECA EXTERNA Layer of delicate connective tissue surrounding the Graafian follicle, external to the theca externa.

THECA INTERNA Thin layer of vascular fibro-elastic connective tissue surrounding the Graafian follicle. Cells produce progesterone in corpus luteum.

THYROID GLAND Endocrine gland found in the neck, which produces thyroxine which in turn is concerned with general body metabolism.

THYMIC (*Hassal's*) CORPUSCLE Small bodies of flattened epithelial cells found in the thymus.

TONSIL A collection of lymphoid tissue; pharyngeal, lingual, and palatine.

TRANSITIONAL EPITHELIUM Stratified epithelium, primarily found in the urinary system. Superficial cells may "balloon" on the surface. Cells vary in shape depending upon whether stretched or relaxed.

TUNICA ADVENTITIA The outer connective tissue coat of an organ which is not covered by a serous membrane.

TUNICA ALBUGINEA Layers of dense fibro-elastic connective tissue surrounding the testes deep to the tunica vaginalis; the inner surface is highly vascularized and known as the tunica vasculosa.

TUNICA INTIMA Innermost lining of the blood vessel.

TUNICA MEDIA Middle layer of a blood vessel.

VON KUPFER CELLS Cells lining the hepatic sinusoids. Phagocytic and part of the reticulo-endothelial system; macrophages.

VASA VASORUM The blood vessels that supply arteries and veins.

VESICULAR Pertaining to a rather light and scattered distribution of nuclear chromatin.

VILLUS Mucosal projection of the intestines and placenta.

VOLKMANN'S CANAL Transverse vascular canals in bone connecting with Haversian canals.

VON EBNER'S GLAND A group of serous glands located in the region of the vallate papillae of the tongue.

WHITE MATTER The thick peripheral layer of the spinal cord composed primarily of longitudinally directed nerve fibers.

ZONA FASCICULATA Area of the adrenal cortex between the superficial zona glomerulosa and deep zona reticularis. Cells line up in parallel rows, separated by sinusoids. Produce hormones concerned with carbohydrate metabolism.

ZONA GLOMERULOSA Most superficial area of the adrenal cortex. Cells in arcades and produce hormones concerned with mineral metabolism.

REFERENCES

Andrew, W. *Textbook of Comparative Histology*. New York: Oxford University Press, 1959.

Andrew, W. *Microfabric of Man: A Textbook of Histology*. Chicago: Year Book Medical Publishers, Inc., 1966.

Arey, L. B. *Human Histology*. 3rd edition. Philadelphia: W. B. Saunders Co., 1968.

Bevelander, G. *Outline of Histology*. 6th edition. St. Louis: C. V. Mosby Co., 1970.

Bloom, W. and D. W. Fawcett. *A Textbook of Histology*. 9th edition. Philadelphia: W. B. Saunders Co., 1968.

Carpenter, A. M. *Human Histology: A Color Atlas*. New York: McGraw-Hill Book Co., 1968.

Copenhaver, W. M., R. P. Bunge, and M. B. Bunge. *Bailey's Textbook of Histology*. 16th edition. Baltimore: The Williams & Wilkins Co., 1971.

Di Fiore, M. S. H. *An Atlas of Human Histology*. 3rd edition. Philadelphia: Lea & Febiger, 1967.

Elias, H. and J. E. Pauly. *Human Microanatomy*. Chicago: Da Vinci Publishing Co., 1961.

Greep, R. O. (editor) *Histology*. 2nd edition. New York: McGraw-Hill Book Co., 1966.

Guyton, A. C. *Textbook of Medical Physiology*. Philadelphia: W. B. Saunders Co., 1966.

Ham, A. W. *Histology*. 6th edition. Philadelphia: J. P. Lippincott Co., 1969.

Leeson, C. R. and T. S. Leeson. *Histology*. 2nd edition. Philadelphia: W. B. Saunders Co., 1970.

Patterson, R. C. and F. N. Miller. *A Graphic Review of Histology*. Washington, D.C.: The Sigma Press, 1958.

Pearse, A. G. E. *Histochemistry - Theoretical and Applied*. 3rd edition. Boston: Little, Brown & Co., 1968.

Pease, D. C. *Histological Technics for Electron Microscopy*. 2nd edition. New York: Academic Press, 1964.

Piliero, S. J., M. S. Jacobs, and S. Wischnitzer. *Atlas of Histology*. Philadelphia: J. P. Lippincott Co., 1965.

Reith, E. J. and M. H. Ross. *Atlas of Descriptive Histology*. New York: Harper & Row, 1965.

Segal, A. H. *Morphology and Anatomy of the Human Dentition*. Chicago: Year Book Medical Publishers, Inc., 1963.

Sicher, H. and S. N. Bhaskar. *Orban's Histology and Embryology*. 7th edition. St. Louis: C. V. Mosby Co., 1972.

Stiles, K. A. *Handbook of Histology*. 5th edition. New York: McGraw-Hill Book Co., 1968.

Truex, R. C. and M. B. Carpenter. *Strong and Elwyn's Human Neuroanatomy*. 6th edition. Baltimore: The Williams & Wilkins Co., 1969.

Wintrobe, M. M. *Clinical Hematology*. 6th edition. Philadelphia: Lea & Febiger, 1967.